Risk, Pregnancy and Childbirth

Over the last hundred years, pregnancy and childbirth has become increasingly safe – yet it is still a site of risk, and a contested ground on which health professionals and pregnant women both face high costs of error. In this context, all those involved in managing pregnancy and birth are expected to identify and mitigate risk: pregnant women are subject to increasing surveillance to ensure the safety of the unborn foetus, and every aspect of childbearing is increasingly medicalised. This publication brings together fascinating social science research to explore the ways in which risk is both created and managed in pregnancy and childbirth. The introductory chapters reflect on the changing social context of childbirth, in particular the medicalisation of both pregnancy and childbirth with development of specialist practitioners, such as obstetricians and midwives who claim to have the knowledge, technology and skills to identify and manage the risks involved. The next three chapters examine the ways in which women's behaviour during pregnancy is constructed as potentially risky – for example smoking, drinking alcohol and taking drugs, and how these risks are monitored and mitigated. The final two chapters of the book address the construction of and responses to both medicalisation and risk in childbirth. Altogether, the contributions represents a valuable insight into the complex world of pregnancy, childbirth and risk.

This book brings together editorials and articles originally published in special and open issues of *Health, Risk & Society.*

Kirstie Coxon is Associate Professor in the Department of Midwifery, Kingston and St George's Faculty of Health, Social Care and Education, London. She is a registered nurse and midwife with a masters degree in Health Policy and a PhD in Health Studies, and has developed a publication profile in relation to risk in maternity care.

Mandie Scamell is Senior Lecturer at the School of Health Sciences, City University London. She is a registered midwife who has a doctoral degree in Social Policy. She has a growing publication profile in risk and midwifery practice.

Andy Alaszewski is Emeritus Professor at the University of Kent and founding editor of *Health Risk & Society*. He is an applied social scientist who has been involved in research on health policy and risk for over 40 years.

Risk, Pregnancy and Childbirth

Edited by
**Kirstie Coxon, Mandie Scamell and
Andy Alaszewski**

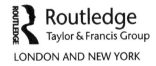

LONDON AND NEW YORK

First published 2017 by Routledge

2 Park Square, Milton Park, Abingdon, Oxfordshire OX14 4RN
52 Vanderbilt Avenue, New York, NY 10017

Routledge is an imprint of the Taylor & Francis Group, an informa business

First issued in paperback 2018

British Library Cataloguing in Publication Data
A catalogue record for this book is available from the British Library

ISBN 13: 978-1-138-29056-3 (hbk)
ISBN 13: 978-0-367-14244-5 (pbk)

Typeset in Times New Roman
by RefineCatch Limited, Bungay, Suffolk

Publisher's Note
The publisher accepts responsibility for any inconsistencies that may have
arisen during the conversion of this book from journal articles to book chapters,
namely the possible inclusion of journal terminology.

Disclaimer
Every effort has been made to contact copyright holders for their permission to
reprint material in this book. The publishers would be grateful to hear from any
copyright holder who is not here acknowledged and will undertake to rectify
any errors or omissions in future editions of this book.

Contents

CONTENTS

Citation Information

The following chapters were originally published in *Health, Risk & Society*, volume 16, issues 1–2 (2014). When citing this material, please use the original page numbering for each article, as follows:

Chapter 2
Editorial: Pregnancy, birth and risk: an introduction
Barbara Katz Rothman
Health, Risk & Society, volume 16, issues 1–2 (2014), pp. 1–6

Chapter 3
'Knowledge is power': risk and the moral responsibilities of the expectant mother at the turn of the twentieth century
Helga Kristin Hallgrimsdottir and Bryan Eric Benner
Health, Risk & Society, volume 16, issues 1–2 (2014), pp.7–21

Chapter 4
'I don't think it's risky, but. . .': pregnant women's risk perceptions of maternal drinking and smoking
Raphaël Hammer and Sophie Inglin
Health, Risk & Society, volume 16, issues 1–2 (2014), pp.22–35

Chapter 5
The risk of being 'too honest': drug use, stigma and pregnancy
Camille Stengel
Health, Risk & Society, volume 16, issues 1–2 (2014), pp. 36–50

Chapter 7
To what extent are women free to choose where to give birth? How discourses of risk, blame and responsibility influence birth place decisions
Kirstie Coxon, Jane Sandall and Naomi J. Fulop
Health, Risk & Society, volume 16, issues 1–2 (2014), pp. 51–67

Chapter 8
Negotiating risky bodies: childbirth and constructions of risk
Rachelle Joy Chadwick and Don Foster
Health, Risk & Society, volume 16, issues 1–2 (2014), pp. 68–83

Chapter 10

Time, risk and midwife practice: the vaginal examination
Mandie Scamell and Mary Stewart
Health, Risk & Society, volume 16, issues 1–2 (2014), pp. 84–100

Chapter 11

Pregnancy, risk perception and use of complementary and alternative medicine
Mary Mitchell and Stuart McClean
Health, Risk & Society, volume 16, issues 1–2 (2014), pp. 101–116

The following chapters were originally published in *Health, Risk & Society*, volume 16, issue 6 (2014). When citing this material, please use the original page numbering for each article, as follows:

Chapter 1

Editorial: Risk in pregnancy and birth: are we talking to ourselves?
Kirstie Coxon
Health, Risk & Society, volume 16, issue 6 (2014), pp. 481–493

Chapter 6

'Why take chances?' Advice on alcohol intake to pregnant and non-pregnant women in four Nordic countries
Anna Leppo, Dorte Hecksher and Kalle Tryggvesson
Health, Risk & Society, volume 16, issue 6 (2014), pp. 512–529

The following chapter was originally published in *Health, Risk & Society*, volume 17, issues 5–6 (2015). When citing this material, please use the original page numbering for the article, as follows:

Chapter 9

Pluralist risk cultures: the sociology of childbirth in Vanuatu
Karen Lane
Health, Risk & Society, volume 16, issues 5–6 (2015), pp. 349–367

The following chapter was originally published in *Health, Risk & Society*, volume 14, issue 2 (2012). When citing this material, please use the original page numbering for the article, as follows:

Chapter 12

Fateful moments and the categorisation of risk: Midwifery practice and the ever-narrowing window of normality during childbirth
Mandie Scamell and Andy Alaszewski
Health, Risk & Society, volume 14, issue 2 (2012), pp. 207–221

For any permission-related enquiries please visit:
http://www.tandfonline.com/page/help/permissions

Notes on Contributors

Andy Alaszewski is Emeritus Professor at the University of Kent and founding editor of *Health, Risk & Society*.

Bryan Eric Benner is a MA student at the Department of Sociology, University of Victoria, Canada.

Rachelle Joy Chadwick is based at the Women's Health Research Unit, University of Cape Town, Cape Town, South Africa.

Kirstie Coxon is Associate Professor at Kingston and St George's, Faculty of Health, Social Care and Education, London, UK.

Don Foster is based at the Department of Psychology, University of Cape Town, South Africa.

Naomi J. Fulop is based at the Department of Applied Health Research, University College London, UK.

Helga Kristin Hallgrimsdottir is Associate Professor of Sociology at the Department of Sociology, University of Victoria, Canada.

Raphaël Hammer is based at the University of Health Sciences (HESAV), Switzerland.

Dorte Hecksher is a PhD student at the Department of Forensic Psychiatry, Aarhus University Hospital, Risskov, Denmark.

Sophie Inglin is based at the University of Health Sciences (HESAV), Switzerland.

Karen Lane is Senior Lecturer in Sociology at the Faculty of Arts and Education, Deakin University, Australia.

Anna Leppo is a Researcher at the Department of Social Research, University of Helsinki, Finland.

Stuart McClean is Senior Lecturer in Health Sciences (Social Anthropology) at the Department of Health and Applied Social Sciences, University of the West of England, Bristol, UK.

Mary Mitchell is Senior Lecturer at the Department of Nursing and Midwifery, University of the West of England, Bristol, UK.

Barbara Katz Rothman is Professor of Sociology at the City University of New York, USA.

Jane Sandall, CBE, is a Professor at the Division of Women's Health, Women's Health Academic Centre (King's Health Partners), King's College London, UK.

Mandie Scamell is Senior Lecturer at the School of Health Sciences, City University London, UK.

Camille Stengel is a Research Fellow at the London School of Hygiene and Tropical Medicine, UK.

Mary Stewart is a Consultant Midwife at Guy's and St Thomas' NHS Foundation Trust, London, UK.

Kalle Tryggvesson is a Researcher and Lecturer at the Department of Criminology, University of Stockholm, Sweden.

Risk in pregnancy and birth: are we talking to ourselves?

Kirstie Coxon

Division of Women's Health, Women's Health Academic Centre (King's Health Partners), King's College, London, UK

In this editorial, I explore the contribution of the recent special issue of *Health, Risk & Society* (Volume 16, Issue 1), and three related papers published in the current volume (Volume 16, Issue 6), and identify themes and concepts which are consistent across these papers. The aims of the special issue were twofold; the call for papers invited articles on the topic of risk in relation to pregnancy and childbirth, and which sought to explore risk theorisation in this field. Looking at these papers as a body of work, I explore the breadth of this collective endeavour, and identify areas which have been researched at some depth, whilst drawing attention to other areas which manage to evade our theoretical gaze. I also reflect on the ways in which these papers have, independently and together, added to the field of risk theorisation, and propose some future directions which might usefully help move beyond the current limits of our enquiry. The combined body of work in these issues represents a considerable resource, and one which makes a clear contribution to contemporary understandings of risk, pregnancy and birth, however I argue that of late, the focus of enquiry has become narrowed, with much of our research providing new evidence from the perspective of relatively privileged women from high-income countries, who have good access to safe, high quality maternity care. The sum of this work is now such that it is possible to synthesise themes across studies and settings, which is valuable to our understanding, but the lack of research amongst women from developing nations, or amongst those with less privilege in high-income countries, means that our resource is incomplete, and fails to do justice to women's broader experience of pregnancy and birth. Developments of risk theorisation are evident in the collected papers; authors have interrogated the positioning of individuals as subjects, and drawn new conclusions about historicised risk, and practices of resistance to risk discourse. I review these developments in this editorial, and also propose that the collection generates many new dimensions to our initial understanding of the 'virtual object' of risk in the context of pregnancy and birth. I conclude by outlining potential new directions and approaches to meet some of the identified gaps in our exploration and theorisation of risk in pregnancy and birth.

Introduction

A recent special issue of *Health, Risk & Society* (16 (1–2)) focussed on risk in pregnancy and birth. This brought together a set of papers with a common theme; each answered a call for articles that explored ways in which risk is understood or constructed by different agents, and sought to extend theoretical thinking about risk in pregnancy and birth. We took as a starting point that 'pregnancy and child birth have become important sites of risk in late modern societies' (Coxon, Scamell, & Alaszewski, 2012, p. 505) and acknowledged the ubiquity of what Lee and colleagues describe as 'the imperative at the individual level to become a risk manager' (Lee, Macvarish, & Bristow, 2010, p. 299).

In this editorial, I review the contribution of the special issue on pregnancy and childbirth, and consider the extent to which the collected body of work adds new understanding to the topical field overall, and to social science understandings of risk in particular. First, I briefly outline recent changes that affect pregnancy and birth from an international perspective to establish a context for this renewed enquiry, and argue that these changes have gradually reframed the ways that risk in pregnancy and birth is constructed from multiple perspectives. I then examine the papers included in the special issue and the three new papers that appear in this edition (Jette, Vertinsky, & Ng, 2014; Leppo, Hecksher, & Tryggvesson, 2014; Wiggington & Lafrance, 2014) as a core body of work. I interrogate the theoretical content and debates within these papers to highlight new insights, with particular reference to a proliferation of 'virtual objects' (Van Loon, 2002) in accounts of pregnancy and birth risk. I identify gaps in the established body of work and argue that this theoretical enquiry has overlooked some important areas in relation to historical discourse, and to understanding intersections of inequality in relation to risk, and it is important to examine why this might be the case.

International focus: current debates in pregnancy and birth

Whilst it is not possible to rehearse here the full extent of international change in relation to pregnancy and birth, some key trends and concerns are important. The division of the globe into low-income regions where birth remains dangerous for women and babies, and regions where women can expect safe, high quality care, is stark; this basic inequity is the focus of the United Nations' Millennium Development Goal Five (Maternal Health), which aims to reduce the maternal mortality ratio by three quarters and provide universal access to reproductive health by 2015 (http://www.un.org/millenniumgoals/maternal. shtml, Renfrew et al., 2014). In high- and middle-income countries, perspectives on birth are also changing; concerns about rising costs, medicalisation, morbidity and variations in care mean that the 'techno-scientific' approach to birth, so long considered dominant, is under concerted attack, and a gradual transformation towards 'scientific-bureaucratic' medicine (Harrison & Wood, 2000) is apparent. Although the practice of obstetrics has been historically resilient to such attacks (see, for example, Arney, 1982; Donnison, 1988), some change is evident; witness, for example, the American College of Obstetricians and Gynaecologists' position paper on home birth (American College of Obstetricians and Gynecologists, 2011); for the first time, this highly conservative professional group is edging towards some level of support from US obstetricians for this practice.

In this respect, the USA lags behind the UK, where there is already established cross-professional support for birth at home and in midwifery units as well as in hospital, and active endorsement of normal birth (NCT/RCM/RCOG, 2007) and vaginal birth following a previous birth by Caesarean Section by both obstetricians and midwives. These initiatives have taken place within a policy environment which is, in rhetorical terms at least, supportive of birth choice for women, and of 'low tech' birthing when women are healthy and well. In 1993, the publication of *Changing Childbirth* (Department of Health, 1993), a policy statement which arguably changed the landscape of birth in the UK by proposing that women should be involved in decisions about their care as a matter of course, and offered women choice (including home birth), control and continuity of care. At a 'witness' seminar held to commemorate the twenty-year anniversary of this policy statement, which has been maintained and even expanded by successive governments, individuals involved in the original drafting joined a panel to discuss its legacy, and to consider the extent to which childbirth has indeed changed. The panel noted that the home birth rate remains static twenty years on, and that the main change has been an increase in birth intervention and surgical birth; this change is certainly not in keeping with the aspirations underpinning the policy, but as one obstetrician commented, what has changed childbirth in England is not the policy framework, but rather the realities of litigation, and the introduction of the Clinical Negligence Scheme for Trusts in 2003 (McIntosh, 2014, p. 28). Clinical Negligence Scheme for Trusts is a 'risk pooling' scheme into which English National Health Service (NHS) trusts pay on a voluntary basis, and can then draw upon in the event of a maternity litigation claim. The amount a Trust pays depends on the level of compliance with Clinical Negligence Scheme for Trusts maternity standards, each of which must be evidenced within Trust guidelines or protocols; discount between 10–30% can be gained by demonstrating adherence to these, including auditing of compliance with guidelines by staff.

The way that these changes are implemented through policy and legislation can be understood within the framework Scamell and Stewart describe as a shift from professional autonomy towards encoded models of governance for pregnancy and birth risks (Scamell & Stewart, 2014, p. 85). These authors argue that clinical governance has become 'a form of collective self-regulation...based on [Harrison and Wood's (2000) concept of] *scientific-bureaucratic* medicine'. This change is directly related to the perceived costs of litigation, as governments and healthcare funders seek to homogenise maternity care by reducing scope for variations brought about by individual clinical autonomy. The historical focus on obstetric practice as the sole source of intervention risk during birth is therefore now outdated; as Annandale (1989) observed in her rather prescient paper, to understand medical care, we need to learn what the lawyers are doing, and how professional practices change because of this.

Scamell and Stewart (2014) explored clinicians' loss of autonomy and the effects this had on their clinical and professional identities, and presented data that showed how, as UK midwives found themselves straitened by both National Institute for Health and Care Excellence (NICE) clinical guidance and fear of litigation (either their own fear, or the sense of a litigation-fearing culture within their employing NHS organisation, or both), women in their care also lost autonomy as choices were downplayed or no longer even offered. Whilst clinical autonomy and the 'techno-scientific' approach to birth may then be weakened, risk governance 'solutions' still close down choice, control and autonomy for women, and the benefits anticipated by detractors of the biomedical model continue to elude us. Rather, it appears that surveillance medicine has merely shifted into a higher gear, capable of instigating what Brown and Crawford (2003, p. 67) describe as 'deep' self-regulation amongst individuals and organisations. In less affluent, middle-income countries however, as Chadwick and Foster (2014, p. 71) remind us, the techno-scientific model is expanding apace; a sentinel indication being that countries such as China, Mexico and Chile report caesarean section rates in excess of 50%, compared to 25% in UK and 32% in US.

What did we know, and what do we need to know?

Health, Risk & Society is a journal with international scope, and risk issues in pregnancy and birth a prime example of a topic with global relevance, yet most of the papers in the special issue refer to research undertaken in high-income countries. Only one paper

(Chadwick & Foster, 2014) came from a country with a developing economy (South Africa), but even so, as the authors acknowledged, the focus was on affluent, educated and mainly white women's' perspectives of pregnancy risk. Almost all of the empirical work in the special issue collection arose from samples of privileged women; the main exception is Stengel's paper, which considered licit and illicit drug use during pregnancy (Stengel, 2014). Stengel opted not to collect demographic data; understandably, her participants expressed a strong need for anonymity, and may not have participated if such information were collected and held by the research team, but Stengel comments that contextual details within women's accounts pointed to marked levels of socio-economic deprivation operating alongside the effects of stigma. In this issue, Wiggington and Lafrance (2014) recount interviews with women who smoked during pregnancy, and again, precise demographic data were not included, but sample description suggests most participants were employed with post-high-school qualifications. Our paper on place of birth in England included a diverse sample in terms of ethnicity and levels of education and affluence (Coxon, Sandall, & Fulop, 2014), although we did not highlight the impact of socio-economic status on birth risk constructions in this article. This does not mean that accounts from women with privileges of affluence and education are not valuable; on the contrary, as these papers illustrate, socio-economic privileges offer little insurance against the complex identity work that women must undertake in becoming mothers. Nevertheless, this collection represents a partial and imbalanced sociology of pregnancy and birth risk with important omissions that obscure the experiences of many women, and this imbalance is certainly replicated in the discipline more widely.

Theorising risk in pregnancy and birth

Each of the papers in our special issue details a particular aspect of how societies and individuals construct and enact pregnancy and birth risk, and the resulting resource, rich in detailed data on lived experiences, certainly builds deeper understanding and establishes links and corollaries across the field. To some extent, the homogeneity of the original samples, which might be considered a limitation of the special issue as a whole, increases the potential for theoretical synthesis across the papers. For example, two papers (Chadwick & Foster, 2014; Coxon et al., 2014) explored place of birth; both used a sociocultural approach, drawing respectively on Lupton (1999a, 1999b) and Beck (1992) and each positioned women as self-regulating risk managers within a risk society. Both papers confirmed the prominence of faith in techno-scientific birthing amongst women who chose hospital labour wards (Coxon et al., 2014) and caesarean birth (Chadwick & Foster, 2014), each echoing Bryant, Porter, Tracy, and Sullivan (2007) and Davis-Floyd's earlier work on this subject (Davis-Floyd, 1994). Each paper also added something new, which is that women described how childbirth involved 'risks of birthing embodiment' (Chadwick & Foster, 2014, p. 80), such as loss of dignity, or public shame. The issues of public and private 'pollution' in birth have been reported before (see, for example, Callaghan, 2007), but the observation that women might seek to control these risks *either* by birthing at home (where home is considered to be private and intimate), *or* in hospital (where hospital is thought to be safe and clean), is new, and points to a deeper set of beliefs about risk and place; the conceptualisation of different venues as 'safe havens', depending on associations with private and public pollution, represents a potential theoretical development. Both papers also speak to the nature of consumer relations within maternity care, and the influence this has on personal control over clinical decisions, and these discussions, again building on earlier work by Davis-Floyd (1990,

1994) and Lupton (1997), point to a new consumer-oriented risk perspective in contemporary health economies.

Across the special issue, authors consistently drew on prominent theorists associated with sociocultural understandings of risk; Beck (1992, 1999), Lupton (1999a, 1999b), Douglas (1966, 1992), Douglas and Wildavsky (1982) and Giddens (1991b) provide the theoretical bedrock for this accumulated work. Within these analyses, sociocultural theories of risk were largely endorsed without a great deal of critical interrogation, which raises the issue of the extent to which such analyses are self-replicating; if we anticipate that sociocultural influences affect risk perceptions, then this is what we are most likely to observe and report. We teach students that articles and research reports are more intellectually robust once the theoretical and analytical position is rendered explicit, but if theory is static then there may be a point where it becomes an artefact, lending credibility but limiting analytical horizons. It seems important to examine whether these approaches still hold explanatory power, and to understand the extent to which our collective work drives theoretical development.

The first paper in the special edition (Hallgrimsdottir & Benner, 2014) certainly challenges our historical understanding of reflexivity and self-governance, and the origins of these concepts. The paper explores the 'moral responsibilities' of pregnant women through published 'maternal hygiene manuals' at the turn of the twentieth century (p. 7), and critiques the notion that self-governance as a response to risk is a late-modern phenomenon. This would not surprise a scholar of Foucault; the architecture of governance has long been in place, but it does present an obstacle to Beck's (1992) risk society thesis, which rests on the concept of 'individualisation' through freedom from traditional structures in late modern societies. As Hallgrimsdottir and Benner (2014, p. 17) argue, '…the pregnant body entered (late) modernity – or the risk society- already hegemonically constructed as a perilous, volatile and hysterical artefact in need of management by a system of expert knowledge by morally responsible actors'. Similar critiques of the logic underpinning 'individualisation' in late modern societies have been proposed by Miller (2005) and Lawler and Lawler (2008); as Miller (2005, p. 48) observes, 'traditional structures' continue to affect women's experiences of motherhood:

> Clearly, changes in the ways we live mean that for many women becoming a mother is no longer regarded as a gender fate. Even so, motherhood continues to be central to the ways in which women are defined, whether or not they actually become mothers. For those who do… their expectations will be shaped by and through expert systems of authoritative knowledge as they negotiate the 'risky' and morally underpinned path to 'responsible' motherhood.

Epistemological orientation of risk theories

Following Lupton (1999a, p. 35), several authors employ one or more epistemological approaches to risk, comprising either realist 'techno-scientific' perspectives, weak constructionist approaches (where risk perceptions are understood to be mediated through sociocultural processes) and 'strong constructionist' or post-structuralist approaches, associated with Foucault's work. In relation to pregnancy and birth risk, it appears to have been difficult to separate sociocultural processes and mediated risk (see Van Loon, 2014 for a comprehensive discussion of mediated and 'remediated' risk) from the impact of surveillance medicine, and self-governance. For example, Hammer and Inglin (2014) document differences in the relative 'riskiness' of smoking and alcohol during pregnancy, and also explore the dangers of attracting moral sanction through failures in self-control that might damage women's identity as 'good mothers' (p. 31). In fact, the observation that sociocultural beliefs about risks become internalised through self-governance and self-regulation is a feature of all the 'special issue' papers, including related papers in this issue (Chadwick & Foster, 2014; Coxon et al., 2014; Hallgrimsdottir & Benner, 2014; Jette et al., 2014; Leppo et al., 2014; Mitchell & McClean, 2014; Scamell & Stewart, 2014; Stengel, 2014; Wiggington & Lafrance, 2014).

This indicates a shared assumption that there is a strong theoretical association between these related perspectives, which might be reasonable given that each reflects macro-theoretical examinations of the individual within society or culture. On the other hand, the originating epistemologies, ranging from objective positivism to post-structuralist constructionism, could not be more different. Does our conflation of these theoretical approaches mean that as social scientists, we have become party to a reduced critical ability to distinguish between these theories, or at least missed an opportunity to explain the relationships that we perceive? It may be that the time has come to further develop Lupton's (1999a) valuable work in this area, on which we rely so heavily, and to conduct theoretically informed work which will help us differentiate and develop macro- and micro-level theoretical thinking about risk in the context of pregnancy and birth. Our current work certainly privileges micro-level 'lived' sociocultural perspectives, and whilst this endows us with valuable empirical data, it perhaps does so at the expense of a concerted effort towards developing more authoritative understanding of macro-theoretical risk perspectives, and applying these to pregnancy and birth.

The proliferation of virtual objects in contemporary accounts of pregnancy and birth risk

A further theoretical observation from the special issue collection is that rather than working from a single conceptualisation of risk during pregnancy and birth, women (and clinicians) are managing a multitude of risks. This is evident from reading across papers, and brings into question our original assertion that: 'In late pregnancy, the main focus of concern, or in Van Loon's (2002) terms the "virtual risk object" is self-evident – risk categorisations are intended to result in the safe birth of the baby' (Coxon et al., 2012, p. 504). Whilst this may be true of clinical risk categorisation, the empirical data in these papers suggests that 'virtual objects' are many and varied, and responses to different understandings of risk are equally so. This is not to suggest that the safe birth of the baby is unimportant to women; on the contrary, this is a central issue, and further, being *seen* to prioritise the future baby over the present self is a core requirement of 'moral' motherhood in the era of intensive parenting. To explore this issue further, it may be useful to consider Van Loon's (2002, p. 54) explanation of risk as a virtual object, and his argument that the focus of risk is always deferred to the future:

> The problem of risk is that it does not exist without representation. By definition, there is no unmediated risk…Its presence is thus always necessarily deferred. Risk is a potential coming-into-being, a becoming-real…the virtual object is not a hypothetical entity; it is real in the sense that it engenders reality, yet at the same time it is not 'material'…the virtual object is being revealed and ordered by…discursive practices and techniques.

Van Loon continues by unpacking different meanings of 'ordering', the first being a Foucaldian idea of ordering by 'classification', or 'principles for putting things in a "proper place", and secondly, a more literal "ordering", which he likens to a Heidiggerian idea of "calling forth" (into being), engendering and enframing' (Van Loon, 2002, p. 55). This insight may provide a premise for the differentiation of sociocultural and self-governance concepts of risk discussed earlier; the classification categories of 'normal, common, expected' and 'abnormal, out of the ordinary, not anticipated', once applied to pregnancy and birth, or to identities of woman or mother, direct attention to where self-governance activities might be focused and practiced. The process of ordering by 'enframing' or 'calling into being' bears closer relation to cultural-symbolic constructions of risk, and the processes by which mediated views become assimilated into 'what is usual here'. In a similar vein, Douglas (1966, 1996) explores symbolic processes of social pollution and discrimination by 'systematic ordering and classification of matter' (Douglas, 1966, p. 44) and through this, creation of categories of uncleanliness as 'matter out of place' (Douglas, 1966, p. 50).

Using van Loon's concept of risk as a virtual object deferred to the future, the papers in our special issue turn out to contain a plethora of virtual risk objects, some of which have several dimensions, and these are summarised here. First of all, there is consensus about the 'safe birth of the baby' as a virtual risk object; this is discussed in Chadwick and Foster's (2014) paper, in Coxon et al. (2014), and by Mitchell and McClean (2014). In this issue, Leppo et al. (2014, p. 525) identify the foetus as symbolic, 'helpless' and hence 'purer' victim (in the context of advice on alcohol in pregnancy), whilst Jette et al. (2014) find the unborn child to be at risk of a range of dangers, if women fail to adhere to the rituals of Chinese medicine during pregnancy and after birth. In each of these accounts, the same logic prevails; the baby is at risk, and supervision or surveillance by experts, along with women's compliance with mainstream medicine (whether Chinese or 'Western') is required to manage these risks. From women's perspectives, the safety of the baby during birth is also threatened by inadequate support on the one hand, or overly interventive care on the other. For example, Chadwick and Foster's South African women interviewees who chose caesarean section considered that usual care for less affluent women (birth with a 'traditional birth attendant') posed a safety risk to the baby. By way of contrast, women who opted for home birth 'emphasis(ed) connection and bodily knowing over biomedical constructions of risk' (Chadwick & Foster, 2014, p. 80; see also Coxon et al., 2014). The 'safe birth of the baby' remains the virtual object, but the threat posed to this depends on the perceived source of the risk.

In the same two papers, women anticipated that they might also be at risk during birth, suggesting that 'safe birth for the woman/mother/self' is a distinct and important virtual risk object for women, one which appears to be neglected in current literature. The sense of being at risk, or that others are not able to appreciate the riskiness of their pregnancy and birth, destabilised women's sense of 'ontological security' (Giddens, 1991a); they no longer *felt* assured of their safety during birth. In these papers (Chadwick & Foster, 2014; Coxon et al., 2014), the anticipated risks women described were primarily medical or obstetric, but also extended to the 'embodied' risks of birth, where birthing is perceived as abject, primitive and shameful, as women lose control of their bodily noises, fluids and functions. A further dimension of the 'safe birth for the woman/mother/self' virtual risk object therefore encompasses fears about the torn or leaking body, and an enduring sense of shame, exposure and loss of feminine identity.

Scamell and Stewart (2014) identified that from midwives' perspectives, women were conceptualised as being at risk of 'failure' to birth within a sanctioned timeframe. These authors outline practices used by midwives, ostensibly to keep women 'on track' and safe from the potential harms of intervention. In this case, the virtual risk scenario, meaning the situation which may incur risk, is a 'birth with intervention', and the propensity for this to lead to complications renders this a separate form of the 'safe birth of the mother' virtual object. A corollary exists between these midwives' perspectives, and that of some women who opt for home birth, but a different interpretation was found amongst women who opt for hospital or caesarean birth (Chadwick & Foster, 2014; Coxon et al., 2014). Amongst these women, techno-scientific birth and medical intervention was understood as a source of rescue from the uncertainties of 'normal' labour and birth, suggesting that the virtual risk scenario here is 'birth *without* intervention', associated in women's accounts with a traditional or non-hospital setting, and with historical narratives of maternal and infant death (Coxon et al., 2014).

Future moral identity as a virtual risk object

A further grouping of virtual objects concerns the construction and performance of moral identities. In several of the special issue papers, there is evidence that women are concerned, or exhorted to feel concerned about, their long-term future identities as 'good' or 'moral' women, mothers and parents. Hallgrimsdottir and Benner (2014) draw attention to virtual risk objects identified in early twentieth century manuals of motherhood, at a time when maternal and infant mortality was a significant risk of birth. For the woman, moral well-being both during pregnancy and for the remainder of her life course was at stake if she did not keep healthy, participate in medical examinations and screening, observe her body for signs of illness and select an appropriate father for the child; the future child's physical health and lifelong moral character was also considered to be at stake. These authors discuss Richardson and Turner (2001) 'citizenship theorisation', and Lupton's application of this theory to pregnancy (Lupton, 2012), showing that for twentieth-century women, '...pregnancy was understood simultaneously as a site through which women could claim some autonomy (and thus citizenship) through exercising responsible choices, and as a site of dependence and vulnerability'(Hallgrimsdottir & Benner, 2014, p. 16). Little has changed in the intervening years; Hammer and Inglin (2014) found women's role as a 'valued repository' for the baby to be undermined if they smoked or drank alcohol, suggesting that the future moral identity is consciously and actively constructed as a virtual risk object within contemporary public health policy and practice. Jette et al. (2014) identify a similar imperative to construct a moral identity amongst Chinese Canadian women. In Stengel's account (2014), drug-using pregnant women found themselves categorised as 'unfeminine' and described their fears of a stigmatised future identity as parents, and also experienced the consequence of their babies being taken into care, if they trusted professionals enough to tell the truth.

Several papers focus on public health issues in pregnancy and birth (Hammer & Inglin, 2014; Leppo et al., 2014; Stengel, 2014; Wiggington & Lafrance, 2014), and each draws to a greater or lesser extent on the Foucaldian concept of biopower, where observation, surveillance and control of the body are understood as 'ways of combining disciplinary techniques with regulative methods' (Foucault, 1984, p. 268). Although Foucault's theses on biopower and governmentality have been criticised as overly deterministic, with little opportunity for free will or reflexivity, Fox (1997, p. 42) argues that Foucault became more interested in reflexivity and 'practices of the self' in his later work, and sought to explore 'how we articulate our bodies and desires within a subjectivity capable of reflection'. Wiggington and Lafrance's (2014) paper in this issue provides an example of this. These authors describe how women who smoked during pregnancy constructed 'smoking for health' arguments to counter the prevailing biomedical discourse, and used these to position their smoking as potentially more beneficial, or at least less harmful to their babies, than sudden cessation might be. Yet, looking at this and other papers, we can see that such resistances are at best partial; pregnant women do not smoke or drink openly, or in public, and Wiggington and Lafrance's participants preferred short telephone discussions over face-to-face interviews, suggesting that they were not comfortable to be 'seen' as smokers. In these papers at least, practices of resistance are performed to limit damage to pregnant women's moral identity, and to counteract discourses of risk objectification, but do not extend past this point; that is, these practices are not used to assert that pregnant women should be able to make autonomous choices about smoking, alcohol or drug use; probably because to do this might attract considerable sanction.

These public health papers also confirm Wiggington and Lafrance's (2014) observation that when pregnant women smoke (or drink alcohol or take drugs), the default assumption is that they are lacking education or information, and the public health solution is to engage, explain and teach women about the risks that they are taking. Once educated, if the behaviour does not change, women are at risk of being considered potentially dangerous (to themselves, to the foetus, to social consensus) (Campbell, 2005) and may be criminalised for their actions, or subject to procedures that may lead to having their children taken into care. Evidence of actions to remove babies from women who drink heavily or take drugs (see Stengel, 2014) point to the dividing line; once classified as non-normal, recidivist or recalcitrant, women are at the same time pregnant, 'at high risk' *and* posing risk, and become 'virtual risk objects' themselves.

Professional moral identity as a virtual risk object

A different variation on the theme of moral identity as a virtual risk object is contained in Scamell and Stewart's (2014) paper; here, midwives' (and, by extension, obstetricians') professional moral identities are at risk if they fail to follow the rules, protocols and guidelines which form the basis of encoded governance. Although guidelines are sometimes justified by organisations on the premise that they are open to interpretation and that professionals may take a different course of action if they can document their reasons and justify this, Scamell and Stewart's (2014) participants were clearly sceptical about this flexibility, and suggested that the reality is quite different. In their experience, clinicians who do not follow guidelines may be considered 'risky practitioners', and subject to sanctions by their colleagues or employer, and may even lose their licence to practice. In turn, and to protect their careers and insurance status, they may consider pregnant women who request 'out of protocol' care to present a danger to themselves as practitioners; a further iteration of virtual risk objectification. As Van Loon (2002) discusses, the technological rationale which identifies particular responses to risk as problematic becomes invisible, and by this process the 'risky' pregnant woman is created as though independent of these logics.

Taken together, these various 'virtual object' formulations of future risk suggest multiple and complex layers of regulatory risk management (and practices of resistance) that individuals, groups and organisations must undertake to maintain physical, psychological and economic safety, the safety of the future baby, and an intact moral identity as woman, mother, parent or professional. This represents a contribution arising from the special issue, and one that might draw collective attention towards boundary work and the ways in which risks are managed, categorised, acted upon or denied by different actors (Abbott, 1988; Bowker & Star, 1999; Gieryn, 1983), and towards work that uncovers the role of media technologies in both representing and creating risk objects (see Van Loon, 2014). The importance of virtual risk objects within the collected papers gives credence to the continued endeavour to explore pregnancy and birth risk through methodologies that reveal individuals' sense-making, although the gap in understanding about how different actors' interpretations of risk at the boundary of interaction or clinical encounter suggests that innovative qualitative methodologies and ethnographic work would make a valuable contribution here.

Ommissions

Focusing on the theoretical and topical contribution from the special issue on risk pregnancy and birth naturally accentuates what has been achieved, at the expense of what is absent or lacking. One key omission arises because most papers, with the exception of Stengel's (2014) article, recount the experiences of relatively privileged women in high-income countries. As well as providing a highly partial account, the theoretical lens of sociocultural risk theory in these papers focuses predominantly on the individual perspective, and neglects the structural inequalities that affect exposure to and experience of risk. In Beck's (1992) and Giddens' (1991a) accounts of risk reflexivity, the individual in post-modernity is portrayed as confident, educated, affluent, informed and able to adopt a position of choice in relation to expert accounts of risk, but this imagined actor quite probably reflects these authors' own privileged status; discursive opportunities for those without privilege and voice continues to be lacking.

In our special issue papers, authors acknowledged that samples for the most part comprise white, educated and affluent women, and therefore allow a relatively privileged voice to dominate, although other 'privileged' voices, including those of obstetricians, health funders and providers, are absent. Without a more balanced view, and one which pays heed to the many inequities of pregnancy and birth risk, we are in effect participating in the creation of a classed and ethnocentric social science of risk in pregnancy and birth. Stengel's (2014) interviews with drug-using pregnant women showed that the risk of a stigmatised identity, not only during pregnancy but extending into future parenthood, was the *main* risk these women faced. This insight is valuable and significant, hinting that some women, by dint of their behaviours, do not have societal licence even to claim the 'virtual risk object' of a safe birth of the baby; further, the experience of invasive surveillance, to which these women were required to subject themselves, increased their sense of a 'non-normal' pregnant identity with the spectre of discipline and punishment ever-present. As Béhague, Kanhonou, Filippi, Lègonou, and Ronsmans (2008) have shown, pregnant women who lack a valued or privileged identity are subject to risks of maltreatment, restraint, poor support and inadequate or substandard care; we are beginning to open these doors, but the overall paucity of evidence from these perspectives suggests our efforts need to shift towards wider inclusion and deeper enquiry into socio-economic inequity. Bourdieu's work provides valuable but underused analytic resources for these issues; for example, the concept of 'symbolic violence' (Bourdieu & Wacquant, 2002) helps to explain how being mistreated or denied resources appears unremarkable to victims, and is merely taken as evidence of 'the way that things are'. As Olofsson et al. (2014, p. 10) note in their call for risk research to be underpinned by intersectional risk theory, 'the production and selection of "empirical" evidence is a highly political process, masked by discourses of objectivity'; we echo their call for exploration of gender, socio-economic status, ethnicity and the attributes of privilege to be central to the ongoing project of risk research in pregnancy and birth.

Whither risk?

A final reflection on the content of the special issue, and the papers included in this volume, comes as a set of questions. The contribution of any paper, or set of articles, forms an incremental development within the field, but also raises issues about the extent of our enquiry. Although these papers represent a valuable resource, in topical and theoretical terms, what remains unclear is whether sociocultural theory helps or hinders the project of better understanding the contemporary role of risk in pregnancy and birth. We have ample evidence of the constraints, discourses and logics which limit women's choice and control, and yet perhaps we fail to imagine what an alternative to 'risk society' might look like. Is it even possible for women, families, social groups, professional cultures, organisations and governments to behave differently in the contexts of shared existing and preceding cultures and histories, or put another way, can any of us think beyond our cultural landscape? Current debates about 'freebirthing' (home birth without professionals in attendance; see Dahlen, Jackson, & Stevens, 2011) suggest that even privileged women do not have the right to elude surveillance and supervision, the irony being that the freebirth 'alternative' so closely resembles the only choice available to women in low-income countries who have no right of access to safe, high quality maternity care, and this brings us back to the starting point of this editorial. Perhaps risk theorists working in the field of pregnancy and birth, and in general health care, might together begin to unpick the human and organisational costs and benefits of regulation and governance in late modern 'risk societies', to consider the opportunities and burdens we might unthinkingly bestow on developing economies, and ask what reach of regulation societies are willing to concede, and what should be considered excessive.

References

Abbott, A. (1988). *The system of professions: An essay on the division of expert labor* (Vol. 1). Chicago, IL: The University of Chicago Press.

American College of Obstetricians and Gynecologists. (2011). Planned home birth: Committee Opinion No. 476. *Obstetrics & Gynecology, 117*, 425–428.

Annandale, E. (1989). The malpractice crisis and the doctor-patient relationship. *Sociology of Health and Illness, 11*(1), 1–23. doi:10.1111/1467-9566.ep10843996

Arney, W. R. (1982). *Power and the profession of obstetrics* (1st ed.). Chicago, IL: University of Chicago Press.

Beck, U. (1992). *Risk society: Towards a new modernity.* London: Sage Books.

Beck, U. (1999). *World risk society* (Vol. 1). Cambridge: Polity Press.

Béhague, D. P., Kanhonou, L. G., Filippi, V., Lègonou, S., & Ronsmans, C. (2008). Pierre Bourdieu and transformative agency: A study of how patients in Benin negotiate blame and accountability in the context of severe obstetric events. *Sociology of Health and Illness, 30*, 489–510. doi:10.1111/j.1467-9566.2007.01070.x

Bourdieu, P., & Wacquant, L. (2002). *An invitation to reflexive sociology.* Cambridge: Polity Press.

Bowker, G. C., & Star, S. L. (1999). *Sorting things out: Classification and its consequences* (1st ed.). Cambridge, MA: The MIT press.

Brown, B., & Crawford, P. (2003). The clinical governance of the soul: 'Deep management' and the self-regulating subject in integrated community mental health teams. *Social Science and Medicine, 56*, 67–81. doi:10.1016/S0277-9536(02)00008-4

Bryant, J., Porter, M., Tracy, S. K., & Sullivan, E. A. (2007). Caesarean birth: Consumption, safety, order and good mothering. *Social Science and Medicine, 65*, 1192–1201. doi:10.1016/j.socscimed.2007.05.025

Callaghan, H. (2007). Birth dirt. In M. Kirkham (Ed.), *Exploring the dirty side of women's health* (pp. 9–29). Oxford: Routledge.

Campbell, N. D. (2005). Drug-using women as criminal perpetrators drug-using women as criminal perpetrators? *Fordham Urban Law Journal, 33*, 2.

Chadwick, R. J., & Foster, D. (2014). Negotiating risky bodies: Childbirth and constructions of risk. *Health, Risk & Society, 16*(1), 68–83. doi:10.1080/13698575.2013.863852

Coxon, K., Sandall, J., & Fulop, N. J. (2014). To what extent are women free to choose where to give birth? How discourses of risk, blame and responsibility influence birth place decisions. *Health, Risk & Society, 16*(1), 51–67. doi:10.1080/13698575.2013.859231

Coxon, K., Scamell, M., & Alaszewski, A. (2012). Risk, pregnancy and childbirth: What do we currently know and what do we need to know? An editorial. *Health, Risk & Society, 14*(6), 503–510. doi:10.1080/13698575.2012.709486

Dahlen, H. G., Jackson, M., & Stevens, J. (2011). Homebirth, freebirth and doulas: Casualty and consequences of a broken maternity system. *Women and Birth: Journal of the Australian College of Midwives, 24*(1), 47–50. doi:10.1016/j.wombi.2010.11.002

Davis-Floyd, R. E. (1990). The role of obstetrical rituals in the resolution of cultural anomaly. *Social Science and Medicine, 31*(2), 175–189. doi:10.1016/0277-9536(90)90060-6

Davis-Floyd, R. E. (1994). The technocratic body: American childbirth as cultural expression. *Social Science and Medicine, 38*, 1125–1140. doi:10.1016/0277-9536(94)90228-3

Department of Health. (1993). *Changing childbirth: Report of the expert maternity group*. London: HMSO.

Donnison, J. (1988). *Midwives and medical men* (2nd ed.). London: Historical Publications.

Douglas, M. (1966). *Purity and danger* (Vol. 2). London: Routledge.

Douglas, M. (1992). *Risk and blame* (Vol. 1). London: Routledge.

Douglas, M. (1996). *Natural symbols* (2nd ed.). Oxford: Routledge.

Douglas, M., & Wildavsky, A. (1982). *Risk and culture: An essay on the selection of technical and environmental dangers* (Vol. 1). Berkeley: University of California Press.

Foucault, M. (1984). Right of death and power over life (from the history of sexuality, Vol. 1). In R. Paul (Ed.), *The foucault reader* (pp. 258–272). London: Penguin Books.

Fox, N. J. (1997). Is there life after foucault? Texts, frames and differends. In A. Petersen & R. Bunton (Eds.), *Foucault health and medicine* (1st ed., pp. 31–50). London: Routledge.

Giddens, A. (1991a). *Modernity and self identity: Self and society in the late modern age* (Vol. 1). Redwood City, CA: Stanford University Press.

Giddens, A. (1991b). *Modernity and self-identify: Self and society in the late modern age* (Vol. 1). Cambridge: Polity Press.

Gieryn, T. F. (1983). Boundary work and the demarcation of science from non-science: Strains and interests in professional ideologies of scientists. *American Sociological Review, 48*, 781–795. doi:10.2307/2095325

Hallgrimsdottir, H. K., & Benner, B. E. (2014). 'Knowledge is power': Risk and the moral responsibilities of the expectant mother at the turn of the twentieth century. *Health, Risk & Society, 16*(1), 7–21. doi:10.1080/13698575.2013.866216

Hammer, R., & Inglin, S. (2014). 'I don't think it's risky, but...': Pregnant women's risk perceptions of maternal drinking and smoking. *Health, Risk & Society, 16*(1), 22–35. doi:10.1080/13698575.2013.863851

Harrison, S., & Wood, B. (2000). Scientific-bureaucratic medicine and UK health policy. *Review of Policy Research, 17*(4), 25–42. doi:10.1111/j.1541-1338.2000.tb00955.x

Jette, S., Vertinsky, P., & Ng, C. (2014). Balance and biomedicine: How chinese-canadian women negotiate pregnancy-related 'risk' and lifestyle directives. *Health, Risk & Society, 16*(6), 494–511. doi:10.1080/13698575.2014.942603

Lawler, S., & Lawler, S. (2008). *Identity: Sociological perspectives.* (1st ed.). Cambridge: Polity Press.

Lee, E., Macvarish, J., & Bristow, J. (2010). Risk, health and parenting culture. *Health, Risk & Society, 12*(4), 293–300. doi:10.1080/13698571003789732

Leppo, A., Hecksher, D., & Tryggvesson, K. (2014). Why take chances? Advice on alcohol intake to pregnant and non-pregnant women in four Nordic countries. *Health, Risk & Society, 16*(6), 512–529. doi:10.1080/13698575.2014.957659

Lupton, D. (1997). Consumerism, reflexivity and the medical encounter. *Social Science and Medicine, 45*, 373–381. doi:10.1016/S0277-9536(96)00353-X

Lupton, D. (1999a). *Risk*. Oxford: Routledge.

Lupton, D. (Ed.). (1999b). *Risk and sociocultural theory: New directions and perspectives* (1st ed.). Cambridge: Cambridge University Press.

Lupton, D. (2012). 'Precious cargo': Foetal subjects, risk and reproductive citizenship. *Critical Public Health*. doi:10.1080/09581596.2012.657612

McIntosh, T. (2014). *Changing childbirth oral history seminar transcript (17 October 2013)*. Nottingham: University of Nottingham.

Miller, T. (2005). *Making sense of motherhood: A narrative approach* (Vol. 1). Cambridge: Cambridge University Press.

Mitchell, M., & McClean, S. (2014). Pregnancy, risk perception and use of complementary and alternative medicine. *Health, Risk & Society*, *16*(1), 101–116. doi:10.1080/13698575.2013.867014

NCT/RCM/RCOG. (2007). *Making normal birth a reality: Consensus statement from the maternity care working party*. NCT/RCM/RCOG. Retrieved from http://www.rcog.org.uk/files/rcog-corp/uploaded-files/JointStatmentNormalBirth2007.pdf

Olofsson, A., Zinn, J. O., Griffin, G., Nygren, K. G., Cebulla, A., & Hannah-Moffat, K. (2014). The mutual constitution of risk and inequalities: Intersectional risk theory. *Health, Risk & Society*, *16*(5), 417–430. doi:10.1080/13698575.2014.942258

Renfrew, M. J., Homer, C. S. E., Downe, S., McFadden, A., Muir, N., Prentice, T., & ten Hoope-Bender, P. (2014). An executive summary for the lancet's series "midwifery." *Lancet*. Retrieved from http://download.thelancet.com/flatcontentassets/series/midwifery/midwifery_exec_summ.pdf

Richardson, E. H., & Turner, B. S. (2001). Sexual, intimate or reproductive citizenship? *Citizenship Studies*. doi:10.1080/13621020120085289

Scamell, M., & Stewart, M. (2014). Time, risk and midwife practice: The vaginal examination. *Health, Risk & Society*, *16*(1), 84–100. doi:10.1080/13698575.2013.874549

Stengel, C. (2014). The risk of being "too honest": Drug use, stigma and pregnancy. *Health, Risk & Society*, *16*(1), 36–50. doi:10.1080/13698575.2013.868408

Van Loon, J. (2002). *Risk and technological culture: Towards a sociology of virulence*. Oxford: Routledge.

Van Loon, J. (2014). Remediating risk as matter–energy–information flows of avian influenza and BSE. *Health, Risk & Society*, *16*(5), 444–458. doi:10.1080/13698575.2014.936833

Wiggington, B., & Lafrance, M. N. (2014). 'I think he is immune to all the smoke I gave him': How women account for the harm of smoking during pregnancy. *Health, Risk & Society*, *16*(6), 530–546. doi:10.1080/13698575.2014.951317

Pregnancy, birth and risk: an introduction

Barbara Katz Rothman

City University of New York, New York, NY, USA

In this introduction, I use my nearly 40 years of work in the area to reflect on the total medicalisation of pregnancy and childbirth that informs even the critical sociology that purports to examine the issue. The risks that are faced in pregnancy and birth are not only the inherent dangers that midwives have worked with across time and space but also those particular risks introduced by medicalisation itself. Medicalisation blinds us to those risks on the one hand, while it blinds us to the skills and knowledge that midwives and birthing women themselves have on the other. The women and midwives researched in these articles show us that in pregnancy and birth, as in most of life, it is not just a matter of 'real risk' versus 'perceived risk' as risk theorists (too) often describe it. There is rather an intelligent balancing of risks, weighing of risks and contextualising of risks. What we see in this issue is a glimpse into the ways in which people intelligently, creatively and determinedly balance risks.

Your editors, each author and the journal itself have done a fine job of exploring the concept of risk, its multiple meanings, uses and abuses. And one imagines that the readership of a journal in *Health, Risk & Society* has thought long and hard about risk.

So, rather than focus on risk per se, I will use my space here to address issues of pregnancy and childbirth – as they are understood in the articles in this issue – and place that in the larger context of pregnancy and childbirth in the contemporary world. But, is it even possible to talk about pregnancy and childbirth in language *other* than that of risk? And 'language' is very much the issue here – these authors use forms of narrative research; discursive constructions dominate discussions of sociocultural risk theories in this issue and in the field at large. The risk consciousness Lupton writes about is found in our words, our talk and our presentations. Our Risk society is a voiced, word-based construction.

So how are we talking about pregnancy and birth?

If you simply google 'risk and pregnancy', you get over 42 million 'hits'. Try 'risk and birth', and you get over 41 million – undoubtedly with some overlap. So no question, pregnancy and birth are understood as having risks, creating risks and being risky business indeed. But not the riskiest of businesses – google 'risk and food', and you get more than two and a half times as many hits, i.e. over 109 million.

That does not feel right somehow – pregnancy and birth are always and everywhere in our world understood as risky, food not so much. A woman announces an early pregnancy and we know the risks of Down's Syndrome, neural tube defects, miscarriage, multiples, prematurity, postmaturity and even stillbirth. Some of us could actually start citing those numbers off the top of our heads – Down's Syndome risks by age, miscarriage by month of gestation and more. It is not just medical personnel who know those numbers – women of childbearing age have had many of those drilled into their heads and anyone who has had a baby has had to sign off on knowing some of those things. And we all, as members of contemporary societies, know factors that 'increase risk' in pregnancy and in birth – drinking, smoking, illicit drug use, being too young or too old, birthing in an unacceptable location, all come to mind and all are dealt with by authors in this issue. And then there are the structural stressors, the race and class issues that we know affect pregnancy outcome, pregnancy risk. There are ever more risks, many of them foods actually – tuna, coffee and even potatoes – have all come and not quite gone as 'risks' in the last quarter century or so.

Outside of pregnancy, food risks are felt less immediate for most of us – I nibble some snacks as I write, sip some tea – Are you worrying for me? Wishing me luck with that? Thinking about the odds of food poisoning? Insecticide exposure? The long-term risks of diabetes, joint pain, heart troubles and cancers that might be flowing forth from the snack choices I am making?

And what about those snack choices? Do they not carry much of the same moral weight that pregnancy choices make – if I tell you it is green tea and carrots, or if I tell you it is a honey chai latte and multigrain crackers with organic almond butter or if I tell you it is a Nestle Iced Tea and Oreo cookies, do I not create different images of myself as a risk-taking or risk-sparing person, even as a more or less 'good' and responsible person? These are, of course, the arguments that Risk-society thinkers have been addressing: the risks we perceive and the risks we take are judged, by ourselves and by others.

It is reasonable to talk about how recent this language of 'risk' is in pregnancy and in birth – but the language of danger, that which we are in risk of, has long been an accepted part of birth, as Hallgrimsdottir and Benner (2014) show. Calling it 'risk' is adding the numbers – sure there are dangers, but precisely what are the odds? That there are dangers in pregnancy and in birth and that they can be avoided or overcome is not news. Dangers and even disasters could happen in the best and healthiest of pregnancies and births. The difference perhaps is that now there is no such thing as a healthy pregnancy – birth, as the obstetricians are fond of pointing out, can only be 'normal' or 'healthy' in retrospect only after the event. There still is an understanding of such a thing as a 'healthy meal' and even a 'healthy diet', but no longer, it seems to me, a healthy pregnancy – the best you can hope for is a low-risk pregnancy.

The pregnant canary in the mine…

If there could be such a thing as a pregnant canary, that is what we had in the coal mine of medicalisation. How can we turn life into a problem of medical management, the body into a site of screening and diagnosis at all times for all purposes? Let us start with how it was done for pregnant bodies – and go from there. Surveillance medicine was, it would seem, born out of pregnancy management, as Hallgrimsdottir and Benner (2014) show. It was early in the medicalisation process, the first of life's stages to be effectively turned over to surveillance medicine. The context, they point out, was three forces coming together: the growth of obstetrics and its grab for professional dominance, the growth of first wave feminism with its appropriation of 'science' and the rise of eugenics, our first science of population management. And what have we now?

A fully realised professional dominance came and went, as the principles of medicalisation were so deeply internalised that the 'doctor' is no longer necessary. People view their own bodies with the medical gaze now, use basic screening tools themselves and turn to practitioners for advanced screening and diagnostic services. Think you are pregnant? Go buy a test. Worried about your cholesterol levels? Want to test with an over-the-counter tester or want to go to a lab or to a physician's office? The key thing is that you cannot know for yourself if you are pregnant or if you are healthy – being late for the first time in your life, feeling that your breasts are tender in a new way, all that means is you should go get tested. Test says no? Try again! Keep testing till the test says what you know to be true. Because you cannot really know, till you have tested. That is the internalised medical gaze. In the early days, the doctor did not trust the woman to know her own body. Now the women do not trust themselves either.

And this now goes way beyond pregnancy: Think you are healthy? How would you know? Your cholesterol could be too high, polyps growing silently in your colon, tiny lumps too small to feel with your hand growing in your breasts, your groin, a shadow on… well, almost anything. Get tested! Why are you sitting here reading this? Something could be growing stealthily in you right now, something that could kill you! Or that something could be your baby. Either way, how could you know without testing? That professional dominance won and surpassed itself, so that it is now not 'doctors authority' but medicalised authority, internalised within, that dominates.

Eugenics as a word is of course entirely out of favour. As a concept and a practice however… well, take a look at the new genetics, at prenatal and newborn screening and at the push to 'have healthy babies'. And more basically, look at the ways that Public Health has moved from an environmentalist approach, making the world safer for people, to a public education model, in which people need to make themselves safer in the world. This too is about population health, much as eugenics was – a good productive society needs good and productive members. And finally we do have the universal acceptance of 'science' as the final word, the truth and, with that, the rather absurd conflation of biomedicine with science, as if the pharmaceutical industries and health and hospital corporations are operating out of science alone. Whatever medicine offers appears to be science: even these authors, looking at the medical pronouncements, and even those without supportive data call them the 'scientific' management of pregnancy. And feminism? Part of what makes the medicalisation of obstetrics to be so very acceptable to educated, egalitarian women these days is its feminisation – women increasingly ARE the obstetricians. What women need to bow down to in accepting medical control is not men, but 'science'.

Risky pregnancy behaviour: policing women

And what is that science? When we read, as Hammer and Inglin tell us, that 'In the late twentieth century, public health experts have identified smoking and drinking during pregnancy as significant public health problems that are harmful to the developing foetus' (2014, p. 22), what are we to make of this? The data on the damage to foetuses of low levels of alcohol are, well, nonexistent might be a good word. The 'alcohol panic' has been nicely researched (see Armstrong 2003), and it is clear that while high levels of alcohol (alcoholic-level high) especially when combined with poor nutrition can indeed cause what is known as 'Foetal Alcohol Syndrome', there is no such data on the damage caused by low levels. But what constitutes 'low' levels? There are no answers and so a kind of decision rule was reached, or what Hammer and Inglin (2014) identify as a 'precautionary approach', advocating complete abstinence. 'Identifying' means labelling, and – sticking just to alcohol for the moment – any alcohol use is labelled as bad maternal behaviour. Kind of. What Hammer and Inglin (2014) also show is that both care providers and women themselves know that an occasional drink has not been shown to harm foetuses and in fact there is no reason to suspect it would. Not surprisingly, better educated, higher status women – women more like their care providers – are given a bit more leeway on this and on occasion take such freedom for themselves. Lower status women are not trusted and know that they are not trusted: abstinence is asked of them.

We see this policing most dramatically in the case of drug use during pregnancy, when on occasions actual police are brought in. While no one is advocating the use of recreational drugs in pregnancy, if the goal was to have healthier women and healthier babies, then a 'harm reduction' model would be in place. Instead, what we see is that women rightly fear punitive responses from their 'caregivers' and from the state. Nine of the thirteen drug-using women Stengel (2014) interviewed feared that their babies would be removed from them when they were born – and they have every reason to fear. Five of them were removed. The long-lasting negative consequences of removing babies from their mothers are largely unstudied – but as one of these women pointed out, there went her plans for breastfeeding. Lower status women know that those assigned with their care are also those from whom they are at risk. Drug use per se is a risk, but clearly so too is being identified as a drug user.

Birth and risk management – managing the risks of the birthplace

The risks of pregnancy drag on for months – women are encouraged to begin risk management long before pregnancy and it continues on over the full duration. Surveillance is inevitably intermittent. But birth takes place over a relatively short period of time, time measured in hours or at most days, not in the months and even years of pregnancy and preconception health.

The rest of the articles in this volume address the ways that birthing women, and occasionally their caregivers, work to manage the risks of medical management. It is those risks, really, not the risks of birth itself that are foregrounded here.

This is perhaps most dramatically true in Chadwick and Foster's (2014) work, comparing women who chose to birth at home and those who requested a non-indicated Caesarean section. What emerges is that for all their differences, both of these groups of women are in agreement that hospitals are not safe places to give birth. Both groups of women are struggling for control: how do you maintain control over your body and yourself at a vulnerable moment? Not by subjecting yourself to medically controlled hospital management. There are two ways these women have found to avoid that: give up on giving birth altogether, become a surgical patient, or give birth, but not under medical management.

Coxon *et al.* (2014) continue in much the same vein – women who choose to birth out of hospital have decided that hospitals themselves are unsafe or, in our language, 'risky' places to give birth. Hospitals are generally understood to be at the ready to provide emergency intervention 'if something goes wrong', but for those women who chose to birth outside of these hospitals, the risks of hospitalisation itself were brought front and centre. Coxon *et al.* (2014) show something interesting – it is not the iatrogenic concerns that those women spoke about, the risks of what is often called the 'cascade of interventions' that follows medical management, leading as it does in over 1/3 of the births to surgical removal of the baby, in what is quaintly called a 'Caesarean section'. The risks they addressed were risks of the hospital itself, what are called, when looking at infections, 'nosocomial' risks: errors that are made when people are managed in what is essentially a factory-like setting, risks of overcrowding, risks of exposure to others and exposure of self.

The rest of the articles show us the ways that women and sometimes their midwives work to manage the risks presented by medicalisation.

In the National Institute for Health and Care Excellence (NICE) guidelines Scamell and Stewart (2014) present, the medical story is that the only way that a midwife can establish that labour is established and can monitor the progress of that labour 'is through an intimate and intrusive action, a vaginal examination' (p. 86). That of course is absurd. Do you really think that an experienced midwife, someone who has attended hundreds or thousands of birth, cannot tell if a labour is established without a vaginal exam? What a midwife needs that exam for is to *document*, not to establish the labour. Those exams are not only 'intimate' and 'intrusive', they are one more interruption and create risks of their own – particularly in hospital settings – and they are one more occasion for the introduction of nosocomial infection. It is managing the management that is being documented; midwives, Scamell and Stewart (2014) show us, use the vaginal exam to create the story that will be most in the woman's best interests, and occasionally in the midwives' own best interest. When those midwives are themselves employees of that institution and 'on the clock', the management of the labour clock is inevitably going to reflect their interests as well as those of the woman being monitored.

If you were given 45 minutes to repair a leaky pipe under a sink, that is it, just 45 minutes in which to get the job done, when would you start the clock? After the tools were laid out, the junk cleared from under the sink perhaps? And if you were being paid by the hour to repair that pipe, then when might you start the clock? When you walked in the door perhaps? People manage timing and clocks in their own interests all of the time. What Scamell and Stewart (2014) found is much what I found about 30 years ago in my own research on home-birth midwives: they were thoughtful about when they measured because they were hesitant to start the clock too early. What they were preventing, what these midwives were trying to minimise, is not the risks of a prolonged labour but the risks of intervening in a labour medically defined as prolonged.

It is not that midwives have no clocks of their own, no ideas about time other than those medicine has established. Not letting the sun set twice on a labouring woman is a long-held understanding in many midwifery settings. It is not that midwives do not have understandings of danger and knowledge about ways to avoid danger – that is precisely what midwifery has been throughout time and across place: the development of a body of knowledge and skilled craftsmanship to navigate the dangers of childbirth.

Nor are women with knowledge of their pregnancies and births, but their own knowledge is systematically disvalued – a pregnant woman who feels her baby moving inside of her, who can – and so many of us have done this – poke and be poked back, turn from side to side to negotiate a sleep position with the foetus within – are said by Mitchell and McClean (2014) to have only 'imagination' and no other way of connecting with their baby.

Mitchell and McClean (2014) follow dominant discourse in their use of the word 'natural', finding it 'ironic' that women think of birth as natural, and prepare for it. Yet, is there anything that is natural for which people do not prepare? Changes in the season? Hunger? Defaecation? Sex? Sleep? Have you ever shopped for just the right pillow? Ever tried to move your bowels at home before you went out for the day? Ever eat food that was NOT prepared? We learn, manage and prepare that which is natural all the time. Women are preparing themselves and using expert assistance, as Mitchell and McClean (2014) show, to avoid medical interventions, which themselves have become the perceived dangers.

What medical dominance has done is not only take over from midwifery and woman's own embodied knowledge of birth, but denied that such knowledge ever existed or could exist. Scientific or 'medical' knowledge is real and authoritative; other knowledge is reduced to 'intuition' or 'spiritual knowing', made all but laughable. But when a baker adds a bit more flour because the dough is sticky, is that 'intuition'? Or is that knowledge based on craft, skill, and deep knowledge of the hands? When a violin maker rejects a piece of wood in favour of one lying next to it that looks just the same to me or to you, is that 'intuition'? Or experience, skill and craft? And when a leading neurosurgeon examines a dozen stroke patients who all present pretty much the same way on all of their tests and feels hopeful about some and concerned for others, is that 'intuition'? Or knowledge based on experience, using a range of senses and information that may not be captured in the tests?

Decision rules

When pregnancy and birth are understood as a series of risks to be controlled, decision rules are in order. You cannot stop and fully research each and every risk or navigate afresh each moment of risk. The first 'decision rule' I learned, as a child was my mother's rule for cleaning the refrigerator: 'When in doubt, throw it out'. The risk of eating food that had gone bad was the risk to be avoided. We were poor – there was enough food insecurity that end of the month, when the check ran out, which meant special treats like noodles for dinner. But we were not so poor that the risk of not-enough-food outweighed the risk of spoiled food. This is the kind of 'risk balancing' people do as they choose to 'err on the safe side'. They look over their leaky boats at both sides, and see which way they are more likely to tip over. Is the drug use the real risk? Or the state's knowledge of that use? Is it the glass of wine? Or the response? Is it going a week or 10 days past your due date, or is it the medical induction? Is it a prolonged labour or a surgical intervention to end the labour?

It is not just a matter of 'real risk' versus 'perceived risk' as risk-theorists (too) often describe it. This is rather an intelligent balancing of risks, weighing of risks and contextualising of risks. And that is perhaps the strongest thing to come through in my readings of all these pieces – the ways in which people intelligently, creatively, determinedly balance risks and come to decision rules.

References

Armstrong, E.M., 2003. *Conceiving risk, bearing responsibility: fetal alcohol syndrome & diagnosis of moral disorder.* Baltimore, MD: The John Hopkins University Press.

Chadwick, R.J. and Foster, D., 2014. Negotiating risky bodies: childbirth and constructions of risk. *Health, risk & society*, 16 (1), 68–83.

Coxon, K., Sandall, J., and Fulop, N.J., 2014. To what extent are women free to choose where to give birth? How discourses of risk, blame and responsibility influence birth place decisions. *Health, risk & society*, 16 (1), 51–67.

Hallgrimsdottir, H.K. and Benner, B.E., 2014. 'Knowledge is power': risk and the moral responsibilities of the expectant mother at the turn of the twentieth century. *Health, risk & society*, 16 (1), 7–21.

Hammer, R. and Inglin, S., 2014. 'I don't think it's risky, but…': pregnant women's risk perceptions of maternal drinking and smoking. *Health, risk & society*, 16 (1), 22–35.

Mitchell, M. and McClean, S., 2014. Pregnancy, risk perception and use of complementary and alternative medicine. *Health, risk & society*, 16 (1), 101–116.

Scamell, M. and Stewart, M., 2014. Time, risk and midwife practice: the vaginal examination. *Health, risk & society*, 16 (1), 84–100.

Stengel, C., 2014. The risk of being 'too honest': drug use, stigma and pregnancy. *Health, risk & society*, 16 (1), 36–50.

'Knowledge is power': risk and the moral responsibilities of the expectant mother at the turn of the twentieth century

Helga Kristin Hallgrimsdottir and Bryan Eric Benner

Department of Sociology, University of Victoria, Victoria, British Columbia, Canada

The notion that 'older' mothers experience elevated risks during pregnancy and child-birth has proliferated since the mid-twentieth century. In this article, we take the contemporary concern with age as a starting point from which to historicise and contextualise the concept of maternity risk. To this end, we examine maternal hygiene manuals (self-help guidebooks on motherhood and pregnancy) published between 1880 and 1920 in Canada, the United States and the United Kingdom. Our analysis of these manuals indicated that pregnancy during this period was presented as a potentially dangerous affair that required constant surveillance by the self (and others) to ensure favourable pregnancy outcomes. A dominant theme that emerged from the manuals was that the expectant mother was morally responsible for mitigating a range of risk factors, including adequate exercise, sleep, fresh air, as well as for choosing an appropriate father and ensuring his health. At the same time, the manuals indicated that the failure to seek out expert advice and take up responsible practices was linked to adverse consequences for the expectant mother's health, and her newborn's health and moral character later in life. We conclude this article by discussing how findings from our historical data can provide an important context for understanding risk discourses around pregnancy as historically specific and culturally contingent, especially with respect to risks associated with maternal advanced age.

Introduction

Recent data on fertility and family patterns in post-industrial nations show that there has been an increase in the number of 'older' women experiencing motherhood for the first time (Statistics Canada 2008, Vézina and Turcotte 2009, OECD 2012).[1] In Canada and elsewhere, this demographic shift has been accompanied by much social anxiety, public debate, as well as medical concern. These concerns have been forcefully conveyed within risk narratives that weave together concerns around the health risks, the ethical and moral challenges, and the social costs of delaying motherhood (Hanson 2003, Gross and Shuval 2008, Silva and Machado 2010, Budds *et al.* 2012) so as to create a dominant conception of late pregnancy as both risky and ethically problematic. The dominance of this narrative of the risky pregnancy of the older mother is particularly interesting given that there is little conclusive evidence suggesting that pregnancy in healthy older women is particu-larly dangerous or that neonatal outcomes differ substantively for older mothers (Carolan 2003, Jahromi and Husseini 2008); indeed, some recent research shows improved developmental and health outcomes of children born to these mothers (Lisonkova *et al.* 2011, Sutcliffe *et al.* 2012).

Scholars have begun to explore how the perseverance of this 'risky' narrative is illustrative of how social contexts are more at play in influencing the biomedical framing of the risky pregnancy rather than the advance of medical knowledge (Markens *et al.* 2010, Burton-Jeangros 2011, McDonald *et al.* 2011, Root and Browner 2011). Issues identified include the power and persistence of normative expectations regarding reproductive timing on our understandings of pregnancy and motherhood and the conflicts between societal expectations regarding the timing of motherhood with other messages around the timing of career and educational trajectories. This work also draws attention to the ways that cultural expectations and norms surrounding pregnancy are imbued with, and embedded within, other cultural and gendered narratives related to the management and control of the female body (Shelton and Johnson 2006, Shaw and Giles 2009, Smajdor 2009, Locke and Budds 2013, Perrier 2013).

In this article, we take a historical perspective to examine the processes through which exaggerated assessments of risk, whether on medical or moral grounds, became discursively attached to the management of pregnancy. To this end, we examine how risk has been historically packaged in narratives of pregnancy aimed at mothers, contained within the pages of maternity 'self-help' manuals in the late nineteenth and early twentieth centuries (1880–1920). As we will discuss more fully in the methodology, we limited our sample to material that was available to Canadian readers, although we did not confine our study to materials published in Canada. Our goal is not only to provide a historical context as to how age plays into normative expectations about risk and pregnancy but also to draw attention to other concerns that have been historically embedded within the range of ways in which we (re)produce and consume knowledge about pregnancy and motherhood. Thus, our aim is to place in a historical context the risk knowledges that currently frame both medical and lay perspectives on pregnancy later in life.

In this, we situate our article broadly within the theoretical risk literature as it has been applied to understanding the medical management of pregnancy. The concept of 'risk' itself, however, is not without theoretical pitfalls, especially as concerns a historical analysis. In particular, the risk society thesis is often understood as essentially coterminous with late modernity (Giddens 1998, Beck 1999) and its application as such within an analysis of documents from the nineteenth and early twentieth centuries would be anachronistic, that is, we would be rendering an understanding of risk from our present state of knowledge that cannot reflect the state of knowledge of the producers and consumers of our historical documents. We therefore adopt the more historicised understanding of risk in the Foucauldian tradition, outlined by Dean (1998, p. 25) as 'a way of ordering reality and rendering it calculable'.

We begin our article by offering some historical context to the elevated risks commonly associated with pregnancy at advanced maternal age by positioning health risks against the backdrop of surveillance medicine. We then discuss briefly some key elements of the historical context (1880–1920) in which the maternity manuals that we examined were disseminated, particularly first-wave feminism and the health reform movements, the medicalisation of childbirth in the late nineteenth and early twentieth centuries and the rise of scientific motherhood ideology. Next, we describe our source material and methods, and then present our results. We end with a discussion on how our empirical findings may challenge the (late) modern theorists who situate pregnancy risk temporally within the risk society, and we also discuss how our findings can help contextualise current understandings of risk associated with delayed parenthood, for both mothers and fathers, as culturally and historically specific.

Context: risk, pregnancy and maternal age

The notion that maternal age is inversely related to healthy pregnancy outcomes is currently so widely accepted that it is (only too) rarely critically scrutinised. It is interesting to note that concern over maternal age has only relatively recently entered the diagnostic vernacular of birth attendants and practitioners. To confirm this trend, we conducted a simple search of 'maternal age' in the PubMed database starting in 1900. 'Maternal age' first appeared in the PubMed database in 1930, with a single article on age and multiparity as determinants of maternal mortality. Eight articles were published on this topic between 1940 to 1950; the number of research articles on maternal age increased in each subsequent decade to 56 (between 1950 and 1960), 613 (between 1960 and 1970), 2331 (between 1970 and 1980), 3068 (between 1980 and 1990), 4862 (between 1990 and 2000) and finally to over 11,000 (between 2000 and 2013). Indeed, early studies of maternal age, such as an Australian study conducted in 1899 (the results of which were later confirmed by Woodbury in 1926), found maternal age to be significantly associated with maternal mortality only among very young mothers (Loudon 1992). In general, there appears to have been relatively little interest in studying the link between maternal age and pregnancy outcomes until the latter part of the twentieth century.

At least two interrelated issues frame this increased interest in maternal age in the last century: the increasing prominence of risk in medical knowledge and practice surrounding pregnancy (see Weir 2006) and the application of surveillance technologies to individuals and populations (Foucault 1973) as a central tool in the management of health through risk assessments. As noted by Lyon (2001, 2003), surveillance technologies have become ubiquitous in our current social and political landscape; more specifically, surveillance has become integral to the practice of modern medicine. Armstrong (1995) locates the rise of 'surveillance medicine' in the early twentieth century. The term surveillance medicine encapsulates important technological, epistemological and ontological shifts in biomedical approaches to managing population health. On the one hand, surveillance medicine refers to the increasing use of diagnostic technology as well as epidemiological and statistical models to create probabilistic understandings of health risks (Bauer and Olsén 2009). At the same time, surveillance medicine has shifted integrally our understandings of health and illness so that health and illness are increasingly interpreted as locations on an ordinal scale: a person who is healthy can become 'healthier' or, conversely, potentially ill (Armstrong 1995, Webster 2002). Thus, surveillance medicine has been successful in problematising 'normal' health by putting healthy populations (and individuals) 'at risk', under constant state and self-surveillance, and subject to the medical gaze through various historically specific disciplinary techniques (for instance, 'healthy' diet and 'adequate' exercise).

In many ways, contemporary practices of prenatal and perinatal monitoring – especially in pregnancies for women at advanced age – illustrate the intersection of risk and surveillance in the practice of modern medicine. Surveillance technologies, on the one hand through risk management techniques, rely on data collection and monitoring in order to improve maternal and foetal care (Chamberlain 2012). From the 1950s onwards perinatal mortality came to be included in surveillance data, and by the 1960s, risk-based perinatal care had come to dominate the institution of pregnancy (Weir 2006).

During this same time, however, risk-based surveillance of pregnancy increasingly rendered foetal health a matter of state jurisdiction (as opposed to medical jurisdiction) which has had profound implications for both public and legal debates around women's autonomy and reproductive rights.

Reproducing risk: nineteenth-century maternity advice and the dangers of pregnancy

As we have argued, our current concerns around maternal age and childbirth are inextricably linked to the rise of surveillance medicine and the attention that surveillance affords to the management of risk in (re)producing a healthy body. During the late nineteenth and early twentieth centuries, however, the increased interest in the medical management of the pregnant body has also to be contextualised within at least two important social and political shifts: (i) the professionalisation of medicine and obstetrics and (ii) the contribution of first-wave feminism to the knowledge and discourse around notions of women's bodies, health and citizenship, nationhood and the uptake of 'science' in aiding women to fulfil their 'womanly' potential as wives and mothers. In addition, both first-wave feminism and the professionalisation of obstetrics occurred in the context of the rise in the popularity of eugenic beliefs as well as heightened political sensitivity around nativist concerns at the turn of the twentieth century in Western Europe and North America. As has been noted by several scholars, eugenics is an important contextual element in terms of understanding social and moral anxieties surrounding pregnancy and birth during this time period in general (Tucker 1998, Lagerwey 1999). Eugenicist and nativist concerns took on a particular significance in the Canadian context. As Valverde (2008b) has argued, racist ideas not only permeated Canadian immigration policy; racist beliefs about the moral character of immigrants, especially immigrant women, were used to justify the need for according higher moral status (and a supervisory role) for white Canadian middle- and upper-class women (Hallgrimsdottir *et al.* 2006, Valverde 2008a, Hallgrimsdottir *et al.* 2013).

The medicalisation and professionalisation of childbirth and the risky pregnancy: Alongside these more general social shifts, this period also captures the ascendance of the profession of medicine and the rise of the medical dominance model (Coburn. 1983, Coburn 1993) which involved, among other things, state regulation in the creation of a monopoly for medicine in the management of health (Coburn 2006). The wide-ranging effects that this shift has had on the management of adverse outcomes in pregnancy and childbirth are well documented (Wrede *et al.* 2009, Benoit *et al.* 2010); of particular interest however is that authoritative claims around skill and expertise in treating pregnant women were central within the larger political project of the professionalisation of medicine in Canada, as well as in other countries (Coburn *et al.* 1983, Fahy 2007).

Professionalisation struggles figure quite prominently in the history of maternity care in Canada (Coburn *et al.* 1983, Wrede *et al.* 2008); in particular, medical professionalisation complemented other nation-building agendas focused on 'civilising' both immigrants and indigenous populations (Jasen 1997). Concomitant with medicalisation was the trend in which pregnancies were increasingly understood for their pathological potential. By the turn of the twentieth century, it was becoming increasingly difficult to distinguish normal from abnormal and pathological pregnancies (Arney 1982). This time period also ushered in a proliferation of domineering technologies in childbirth management such as forceps and operative intervention; expert systems of medical knowledge were increasingly placing childbirth in the domain of (male) obstetric professionals (Arney 1982, Leavitt 1987, Conrad 1992). In addition, as argued by Riessman (1983), women were also active participants in the medicalisation of childbirth in several ways. Women during this period sought relief from the pain of childbirth, as can be inferred from the popularity of morphine during childbirth, a drug promising women a 'twilight sleep' during labour. In addition, the declining fertility rate for women in middle and upper classes made pregnancies rarer events; it follows that the risk of foetal death became a growing concern (Riessman 1983). Finally, the *perception* of the effectiveness of obstetrics by both the public and the medical community influenced the increased uptake of medical and scientific management of childbirth (Smith-Rosenberg and Rosenberg 1973, Arney 1982, Leavitt 1987).

At the same time as asserting their dominance in the management of childbirth over midwives, childbirth was also a site through which physicians could claim expertise and authority *vis a vis* religious interventions in the care of pregnant women (Leavitt 1987). In Canada, the dominant Anglican and Catholic churches proscribed against surgical intervention in childbirth for the purposes of saving the mother's life as morally wrong; in claiming the right to diagnose and intervene, as well as at times to prevent pregnancy, physicians were thus pushing back not only on midwives but also on the Church's proscriptions (McLaren 1978, Backhouse 1983).

Health reform and first-wave feminism. Our time period of interest predates both the rise of surveillance medicine and its accompanying focus on risk management in pregnancy. Nonetheless, the time period has several features that make it of interest for scholars interested in understanding the social processes around which pregnancy began to be primarily understood as a risky endeavour. For instance, it is during these years that health reform movements in Canada as well as the United States emerged and flourished (Richardson 1989). These movements emphasised the improvement of public health through prevention and hygiene (Szreter 2003) while also linking public health with other significant national attributes related to modernity and progress; in this, health of the family (and by extension society) became attached to notions of the responsible exercise of citizenship (Crawford 1994). Another important focus of public health reform efforts was in public education, often through medical and health manuals aimed at and distributed to lay audiences. Women were a central target of these efforts for a range of reasons, but particularly due to the importance of maternalist feminist ideas for shaping the strategies and activities of a range of political and social movements in the public sphere during this time (Morantz 1977, Koven and Michel 1990, White 2002, Hallgrimsdottir *et al.* 2013).

Just as childbirth at the turn of the twentieth century was increasingly becoming subject to the medical gaze and an arena dominated by institutional, specialised knowledge, Apple (1995) has noted that this period was also marked by a proliferation of scientific advice aimed specifically at women to manage the various periods in their lives. This 'ideology of scientific motherhood' (Apple 1995) emphasised that women were responsible for both their own health and the health of their families while at the same time incapable of fulfilling this responsibility. The ideas associated with scientific motherhood were intertwined with maternalist ideologies, described by Michel and Koven (1990) as ideas that raised and glorified women's roles as mothers and attributed the capacity to mother with certain characteristics that rendered women both suited for (while at the same time obligated to) exercise citizenship in the public sphere. Specifically, women's capacity 'to mother' was associated with moral character, care and nurturance (Plant and Van Der Klein 2012). These discourses were presented and disseminated in a range of ways, but perhaps most importantly in the form of childcare manuals produced by doctors, scientists, nurses, advice columns and letters to the editor in women's magazines, and also home economics classes offered at various stages of women's education (Apple 1995). Motherhood no longer relied on women's 'natural' or 'womanly' instincts: All areas of motherhood and preparation for childbirth were in need of expert instruction and management (Pierce 2008).

In essence, the era during which our study is situated is significant in Canada. This is a period of intense and accelerated campaigns to medicalise pregnancy when expertise and authoritative claims of doctors around the management of the pregnant body formed an important part of the processes through which medicine professionalised and gained dominance; in addition, normative constructions of pregnancy were linked during this period to larger historical and cultural projects of modernity, progress and the exercise and responsible practice of citizenship. While women were being educated as responsible creators and managers of the pregnant body, they were also told to delegate the authority in the management of the pregnant body to experts; our article draws on data that captures these competing narratives.

Methods

In this article, we draw on data drawn from our reading of motherhood health manuals published between 1880 and 1920. We searched the HathiTrust digital library, currently one of the largest repositories for digitised archival material. In order to cast the net as wide as possible, we utilised broad search terms in the initial search: 'maternity,' 'mothers,' 'motherhood,' 'moral education,' 'childrearing,' 'hygiene' and 'pregnancy'. We then narrowed down the material in two ways: to material that would have been available to Canadian audiences, produced specifically for consumption by (potential) mothers. We also excluded all manuals and advice books that were specifically affiliated with religious organisations or alternative therapies such as homeopathy in order to limit our sample to mainstream medical advice. These limits resulted in an overall sample size of 14 manuals.

We employed a modified version of critical discourse analysis (Fairclough *et al.* 2011) that involved three considerations: thematic analysis and identification of codes with attention to word choice, use of metaphors, as well as more explicit features of the language used in informing women about maternity and childbirth; attention to the intended audience and possible power relations between this audience and the authors of the guidebooks; and the historically and contextually specific meanings and forms of 'risk'. Within each manual we searched for discussions and passages referring to the health and well-being of mothers and babies with particular attention to the notion of 'risk'. The term 'risk' did not occur frequently. We defined 'risk' during pregnancy and childbirth as anything imputing not only *adverse* but also *preventable* consequences that could be linked to the conduct of (expectant) mothers and their attending carers; in addition, structural and systemic sources of risk (for instance, environmental conditions) were also considered. Additional emphasis was placed on passages that included reference to childbearing age for both parents. Analysis of the archival material was an iterative process whereby codes were generated independently by both authors and then verified by each author independently. These preliminary codes were then ordered into two meta-themes: 'risk' and 'moral responsibility'. We imported our source material into *DeDoose*, a qualitative analytical software package. We present below an overview of the findings, followed by a discussion on the two emergent themes of risk and morally responsible choices.

Findings

Overview

We identified two significant and mutually supportive themes in the discussions around pregnancy and health found within the motherhood manuals that we examined: risk and (moral) responsibility. It was necessary for the mother (but not the father) to be morally responsible for not only knowing the risks and dangers but also acting against them through morally responsible conduct. To this end, the pregnant woman's conduct was exclusively governed by invoking distinctly moral directives aimed against averting possible – and avoidable – dangers. The authors of these manuals positioned themselves as highly authoritative and scientific, and made claims largely informed by clinical encounters and experiential knowledge. The health and well-being of the mother and child were generally emphasised while the foetus was not ascribed the status of a person and did not attract concern in or of itself but more as a means to an end, the healthy baby. While the possibility of pregnancy in 'older' women was thought to decline with women's advancing age, the pregnancy itself was not in general constructed as more or less risky event for older as compared to younger women. However, mothers were often positioned as responsible agents for mediating collective risks to the human species through, among other things, being responsible for selecting suitable fathers for on account of the hereditability of their moral, physical and mental character.

In the manuals, women were invariably addressed in the third person, in some cases referred to at specific life stages through phrases such as 'the young girl', 'the young wife', 'the spinster' and 'the mother'. Some manuals included a brief summary of the author's qualifications while others did not mention their qualifications beyond being medical doctors. The manuals presented expertise covering the selection of husbands and mandates on women's conduct in a variety of areas familiar to those appearing in more modern manuals such as dietary modification, advice on resting, when and how to exercise, sleeping, clothing, bathing, the importance of surrounding herself in atheistically pleasing environments and thinking pleasant thoughts. Some manuals placed particular emphasis on women's tendency to be hysterical before, during and following pregnancy, which in turn was linked to increased risks of miscarriage (as discussed below) as well as birth defects.

Maternal age, childbearing risk and fertility

The maternal manuals in our study mostly associated a woman's fertile period with her menstrual cycle. Women's reproductive potential was thought to diminish generally after age 45 or 50. Most manuals made no specific reference to the upper age range in which women were fertile. In all, women's period of greatest fertility was described as being in her early to mid-twenties. Scharlieb (1919) indicated that between the ages 20 and 25 women were most fertile, noting only that childbearing becomes comparatively rare in the years leading to the menopause. Kellog (1886, pp. 294–295) suggested that the earliest age to marry was not before 20 or 22 because she had not developed physiologically before this period, noting also that populations in the East, the interior of Africa and Italy reflect a high degree of 'physical, mental and moral degeneracy' that can be attributable to mothers' younger – not older – age.

Of the 14 sources included in this study, only one mentioned adverse health outcomes in childbearing at advanced age. *The Physical Life of Women* (Napheys 1890) associated age with miscarriage and adverse mental health in children; firstborns were highly prized yet prone to be lost through miscarriage on account of the hysterical pregnant woman:

> A woman who marries at forty is very much disposed to miscarry; whereas, had she married at thirty, she might have borne children when older than forty. As a mother approaches the end of her child-bearing period, it is likely that she will terminate her career of fertility with a premature birth. The last pregnancies are not only most commonly unsuccessful, but there is also reason to believe that the occurrence of idiocy in a child may be associated with the circumstance of its being the last-born of its mother. It has been asserted, in this connection, that men of genius are frequently the first-born. First pregnancies are also fraught with the danger of miscarriage, which occurs more often in them than in others, excepting the latest. A woman is particularly apt to miscarry with her first child, if she be either exceedingly nervous or full-blooded. (Napheys 1890, p. 192)

Word choice, when describing woman's declining fertility later in life, sometimes invoked imagery of a dying or decaying body to explain this emphatically 'natural' and biological decline. For instance, in *The Ladies' Guide,* Kellog (1886) claimed that when a woman reached 45 her ovaries underwent a 'remarkable degenerative change' as it 'begins to shrivel... a few months later it is still more shrunken; and after the cessation of the menses it often becomes so shriveled as to be scarcely recognizable' (p. 369). Another source, *The Diseases of Women* (Bland-Sutton and Giles 1906), described cessation of menstruation as being 'associated with excessive losses of blood at the periods – the last convulsions of a dying function' (p. 301). *The Diseases of Women* (Bland-Sutton and Giles 1906) also stated that at menopause it was quite possible for a woman to believe she was pregnant, but that this is likely to be an 'erroneous suspicion' because 'women would rather persuade themselves that they are with child than suppose they are feeling the consequences of growing old' (pp. 302–303).

Responsibilities of the pregnant woman

As we have noted, the dominant theme in the maternity manuals that we examined was that a mother must be morally responsible not only for knowing the risks and dangers but also acting on them. The following example is illustrative of the concept described above with also a typical depiction of how 'risk' was employed in the literature of this time. From the introduction to *The Wife's Handbook* (Norman 1914), the text states that a young wife must be taught how to manage her health in early marriage, the most important period of her life:

> [The young wife must be retrained from] the popular ignorance in which she may have been reared... There may be many women who are fit candidates for matrimony... but who are not fit physically to risk becoming mothers... The manifold duties [as wives and mothers] pertaining to these important trusts can only be performed when all the great but simple laws of health are obeyed. 'Knowledge is power.' (Norman 1914)

Women were also instructed to seek the most medically advanced screening technology which, during this historical period, was limited to mandates of regular physical examinations by her physician and, in some sources, urine tests for albumin. Ongoing self-monitoring was encouraged for feelings of nausea, fatigue, pain or uterine bleeding; in the event such a symptom occurred, she was to summon her physician at once.

Sexual activity and dangerous thoughts of the pregnant woman

Most of our sources problematised sexual intercourse during pregnancy. Some gave specific maternal age ranges wherein it was most dangerous, others pronounced that the harmful consequences to mother and child were certain or very likely: 'no woman can submit to such abuse [intercourse] *without injury to herself* and *danger to her offspring'* (Johnson 1889, pp. 52–53; emphasis in the original). Risks associated with sexual activity include idiocy in the child, miscarriage, deformities and damage to the nervous system of the mother.

Several manuals identified masturbation as perverse, a moral vice and directly harmful to the mother. Masturbation was not directly tied to health outcomes in children, but this could be inferred on account of the linkage of heredity of parental characteristics that were generally described as being able to be passed on to the children. This was the case for both mother and father, in language associated with modern conceptions of 'risk' through word choice. To illustrate this, in *The Physical Life of Women* (Napheys 1890), an otherwise clinical and scientifically presented account of womanhood markedly departs to suggest that 'infants are *often* born with various marks and deformities corresponding in character with objects which made a vivid impression on the maternal mind during pregnancy… The child may [also] be affected by maternal impressions acting through the mother's milk' (pp. 196–197; emphasis in the original). All of the manuals that we examined suggested that the deviant sexual conduct and thoughts of the pregnant mother were dangerous to both the pregnancy and to the mother.

Role of mother in assessing the father's health and age

The manuals emphasised that the father's state of health was potentially harmful not only to his children but also to the mother as well as subsequent children that might be fathered upon remarriage to another man. *Advice to a Wife* (Chavasse 1882) is unable to specify the precise way in which the father's ill-health may affect his offspring; it is mysterious but highly probable:

> [A] husband who is not in the enjoyment of good health is not prepared to transmit a good constitution to his children. Although the mother may herself be healthy, she may have imposed upon her the task of rearing children blighted with disease from the very moment of conception… in some mysterious manner the constitution of the wife is modified by that of the husband, probably through the influence of the child during pregnancy, so that her own health may suffer to a greater or less degree as well as that of the child. She should also recollect that the impression thus made on the constitution is ineffaceable, so that though the feeble husband should die and a subsequent marriage be with a healthy man, the resulting offspring might still be affected by the feebleness of the former husband. (pp. 302–303)

The *Ladies' Guide* (Kellog 1886) specified that a responsible young wife should only marry younger men, slightly older yet close to her own age, or else she risked bringing sickly and unhappy children into this world:

> Occasionally, far too frequently in fact, the good sense of society is shocked by a matrimonial union between a blooming young girl and some infirm octogenarian whose only charm is the possession of a large fortune. The children of such a marriage, if it is a fruitful one, are cursed by the results, as well as the parents. The old, unhappy faces of such little ones are really sad to look upon. They are certain to die early, and their premature death is, in most cases, a happy event, both for themselves and the world. Many times scrofula and consumption [both terms for tuberculosis] make their existence a curse to themselves and a burden to others, so

that death comes as a grateful release... As a rule, the husband should be one or two years older than the wife, but the difference should not exceed eight or ten years in favor of the husband. (pp. 298–299)

Discussion

In the manuals we examined, being an older mother was not highlighted as a particular area of danger or risk. In fact, advanced maternal age was found to be a risk factor during pregnancy and childbirth in only one of the primary sources examined in this study. However, these manuals did highlight the role of the father in mitigating the risks of pregnancy. As we noted, the surveillance of pregnancy risks in the twentieth century has largely been aimed at mothers themselves, as responsibilised agents of their own health and that of the embryo, foetus and child. While on the one hand the medical interest in fathers at this time could be understood to construe a shared responsibility for ensuring a healthy pregnancy, it is worth noting that in the material that we examined the selection of an appropriate husband and potential father was a woman's responsibility. This is particularly interesting given women's economic and political dependence on men during this time. Recent citizenship theorisation (Richardson and Turner 2001, Lupton 2012) has examined the central role of sexuality and reproduction to women's historical and contemporary claims to citizenship; in the manuals that we examined, pregnancy was understood simultaneously as a site through which women could claim some autonomy (and thus citizenship) through exercising responsible choices, and as a site of dependence and vulnerability.

The references to paternal age (and, more specifically, to the dangers involved in unions where the father is considerably older than the mother) are particularly interesting. While there has been significantly less interest in examining advanced paternal age as a risk factor in adverse perinatal outcomes, investigations appear to have dramatically increased very recently, corresponding with genetic technology developments. Advanced paternal age has been found to be associated with a variety of health outcomes on par with – and exceeding – those traditionally associated with women's age, including increased risk for children born with Down's syndrome (Fisch et al. 2003) and psychiatric disorders such as bipolarism (Frans 2008) and schizophrenia (Torrey et al. 2009). At the same time, recommendations in the medical community for perinatal screening based on paternal age have not been as widely implemented as they have been for women (Conti and Eisenberg. 2013). While outside the scope of this article, it is thus worth considering how the statistical, scientifically derived risk evaluations that drive policy recommendations for perinatal risk are also deeply inscribed by gendered and highly normative expectations regarding reproductive timing.

Our findings also offer a foundation for contextualising more modern constructions of risk during pregnancy. It is a widely held belief in society at present that pregnancies are, in general, more hazardous, requiring increasingly responsible conduct by (potential) mothers, accompanied by increased (and increasing) anxieties, and certainly riskier having been informed by modern, scientifically calculated medical authority (Lupton 2012). Lupton has written on pregnancies in late modern risk society extensively, pointing to the expert systems of knowledge and strategies mandating self-governance that have proliferated around pregnancy today at a greater scale than in previous eras; this phenomenon has been accompanied by a rise in risk-related knowledges and the various modern technologies employed in pregnancy management. However, a critical examination of the construction of risks and dangers associated with pregnancy at the turn of the twentieth century shows that, through specific, historically situated strategies, the pregnant body entered (late) modernity – or the risk society – already hegemonically constructed as a perilous, volatile and hysterical artefact in need of management by a system of expert knowledge by morally responsible actors. Our limited findings certainly challenge the risk society thesis that reads the management of pregnancy through risk discourses as a late modern project. At the very least, our findings offer an anchoring point for questioning how one might evaluate the extent to which pregnancy is in some way the target of increased or accelerating risk at present.

In all, the responsibilising discourses found in our source material from the turn of the twentieth century appear analogous to more modern forms of responsibilising discourses commonly associated with the management of pregnancy in advanced liberal societies (Shuttleworth 1993/1994, Hays 1996, Ruhl 1999). Whereas there are constants such as recommendations around diet, fresh air and exercise, other forms (such as carriage riding that appears as a risk in several manuals) have been updated to risky transportation technologies of today – for instance, there is currently no gestational period of 'zero risk' for travel by *airplane*. And while a century ago women were encouraged to subject themselves to urine tests and comparatively rudimentary physical exams aimed at determining whether they were indeed pregnant at all, women today are active consumers of home pregnancy tests and the latest in clinical antenatal screening technologies that include amniocentesis and even home ultrasound equipment. The scientific management and responsibilisation of pregnancy and motherhood has thus proliferated ever since the nineteenth century, among other various dominant disciplinary techniques in societies at the turn of the twentieth century.

Conclusion

A historical perspective on pregnancy risks and the moral responsibility of the pregnant mother provides a critical lens that allows us to cast doubt on the axiomatic assumptions surrounding risk and the 'older mother'. More critically, historicising the notion of the risky pregnancy reveals how medical as well as lay concerns with 'older mothers' are certainly more reflective of other social anxieties surrounding reproduction than of advancements in biomedical knowledge.

There are, from our findings, two, likely non-coincidental, observations that can be made about historical and contemporary anxieties about pregnancy and childbirth. When maternal age became part of the diagnostic vernacular of birth practitioners, it was laid on top of pre-existing understandings of pregnancy as not just dangerous, but also as a focal point for the regulation, control and the (self-)disciplining practices of women. This occurred during a time when women were expanding their autonomy and control over their bodies, through, for instance, claiming political membership (through suffrage) and an authoritative voice in public discourse (through, among other things, the purity and temperance movements, as well as claiming a stake in eugenic debates and anti-immigrant politics). Currently, delaying motherhood is one of the few ways in which Canadian women can currently mitigate the high opportunity costs associated with childbirth: in other words, the 'older mother' represents simultaneously the normal (modal) and the abnormal (other). Censuring the older mother thus increasingly implies censuring an ever increasing number of childbearing women, but in particular those mothers whose access to higher educations and higher incomes presumes a certain amount of 'choice' when it comes to reproduction.

These links – both historically and in the present day – between responsibilisation, risk, reproductive choice and autonomy – suggest that understanding the notion of maternity risk requires conceptual language that goes beyond both 'risk society' and responsibilisation perspectives. In particular, Bacchi and Beasley (2002) have used the concept of embodied and sexual citizenship to analyse the complex ways in which power is inscribed through and within legislation aimed at controlling reproduction (Bacchi and Beasley 2002). In their writing, they suggest that considering the 'fleshiness' of citizenship highlights how values of autonomy and dependence are assigned onto procreative and non-procreative bodies. More specifically, procreative bodies are assigned a lesser value as citizens because they are seen to be 'controlled by' their bodies instead of being 'in control' of their bodies. In this way, the discussions of maternity risks and the concomitant discourses of responsibilisation, today and at the turn of the nineteenth century, can be seen to both signal and cement the dependence of the procreative (female) citizen.

Note

1. Canadian women's mean age at first birth is between 27 and 28, an increase of nearly 4 years between the years 1970 and 2009 (OECD 2012).

Archival sources

Ballantyne, J.W., 1914. *Expectant motherhood: its supervision and hygiene*. Toronto, ON: Cassell & Company.

Bishop, H.D., 1910. *Motherhood: a manual on the management of pregnancy*. Cleveland, OH: Rose Publishing Company.

Bland-Sutton, J. and Giles, A.E., 1906. *The diseases of women*. 5th ed. With 129 illustrations. London: Rebman Limited.

Capp, W.M., 1891. *The daughter, her health, education and wedlock*. Philadelphia, PA: F.A. Davis.

Chavasse, P.H., 1882. *Advice to a wife on the management of her own health and on the treatment of some of the complaints incidental to pregnancy, labour, and suckling with an introductory chapter especially addressed to a young wife*. Toronto, ON: Willing & Williamson.

Johnson, I.D., 1889. *Counsel to parents, and how to save the baby*. Kennett Square, PA: I.D. Johnson.

Kellog, J.H., 1886. *Ladies' guide in health and disease: girlhood, maidenhood, wifehood, motherhood*. Des Moines, IA: W.D. Condit.

Napheys, G., 1890. *The physical life of woman: advice to the maiden, wife, and mother*. Toronto, ON: Maclear & Company.

Norman, R., 1914. *The wife's handbook*. Menasha, WI: G. Banta.

Saur, P., 1888. *Maternity, a book for every wife and mother*. Chicago, IL: L. P. Miller & Company.

Scharlieb, M., 1919. *The welfare of the expectant mother*. Toronto, ON: Cassell and Company.

Scovil, E., 1896. *Preparation for motherhood*. Philadelphia, PA: Henry Altemus.

Slemons, J.M., 1919. *The prospective mother: a handbook for women during pregnancy*. New York: D Appleton and Company.

West, J.D., 1887. *Maidenhood and motherhood (or ten phases of woman's life)*. San Francisco, CA: Law, King & Law.

References

Apple, R.D., 1995. Constructing mothers: scientific motherhood in the nineteenth and twentieth centuries. *Social history of medicine*, 8 (2), 161–178.

Armstrong, D., 1995. The rise of surveillance medicine. *Sociology of health & illness*, 17 (3), 393–404.

Arney, W.R., 1982. *Power and the profession of obstetrics*. University of Chicago Press.

Bacchi, C.L. and Beasley, C., 2002. Citizen bodies: is embodied citizenship a contradiction in terms? *Critical social policy*, 22 (2), 324–352.

Backhouse, C.B., 1983. Involuntary motherhood: abortion, birth control and the law in nineteenth century Canada. *Windsor YB access just*, 3, 61.

Bauer, S. and Olsén, J.E., 2009. Observing the others, watching over oneself: themes of medical surveillance in post-panoptic society. *Surveillance & society*, 6 (2), 116–127.

Beck, U., 1999. *World risk society*. Cambridge: Polity Press.

Benoit, C., *et al.*, 2010. Medical dominance and neoliberalisation in maternal care provision: the evidence from Canada and Australia. *Social science & medicine*, 71 (3), 475–481.

Budds, K., Locke, A., and Burr, V., 2012. Risky business. *Feminist media studies*, 13 (1), 132–147.

Burton-Jeangros, C., 2011. Surveillance of risks in everyday life: the agency of pregnant women and its limitations. *Social theory & health*, 9 (4), 419–436.

Statistics Canada., ed., 2008. Children of older first-time mothers: their health and development *Children and youth series papers*. Ottawa, ON: Statistics Canada.

Carolan, M., 2003. The graying of the obstetric population: implications for the older mother. *Journal of obstetric, gynecologic, & neonatal nursing*, 32 (1), 19–27.

Chamberlain, J.M., 2012. *The sociology of medical regulation*. Dordrecht: Springer.

Coburn, D., 1993. State authority, medical dominance, and trends in the regulation of the health professions: the Ontario case. *Social science & medicine*, 37 (2), 129–138.

Coburn, D., 2006. Medical dominance then and now: critical reflections. *Health sociology review*, 15 (5), 432–443.

Coburn, D., Torrance, G.M., and Kaufert, J.M., 1983. Medical dominance in Canada in historical perspective: the rise and fall of medicine? *International journal of health services*, 13 (3), 407–432.

Conrad, P., 1992. Medicalization and social control. *Annual review of Sociology*, 13, 209–32.

Conti, S.L. and Eisenberg, M.L., 2013. Paternal aging and increased risk of congenital disease, psychiatric disorders, and cancer. *In*: D.T. Carroll, ed. *Paternal influences on human reproductive success*. Cambridge University Press, 93–101.

Crawford, R., 1994. The boundaries of the self and the unhealthy other: reflections on health, culture and AIDS. *Social science & medicine*, 38 (10), 1347–1365.

Dean, M., 1998. Risk, calculable and incalculable. *Soziale welt*, 49, 25–42.

Fahy, K., 2007. An Australian history of the subordination of midwifery. *Women and birth*, 20 (1), 25.

Fairclough, N., Mulderrig, J., and Wodak, R., 2011. Critical discourse analysis. *In*: T.A. Van Dijk, ed. *Discourse studies: a multidisciplinary introduction*. Thousand Oaks, CA: Sage, 357–378.

Fisch, H., *et al.*, 2003. The influence of paternal age on Down syndrome. *The journal of urology*, 169 (6), 2275–2278.

Foucault, M., 1973. *The birth of the clinic: an archaeology of medical perception*. New York: Vintage.

Frans, E.M., *et al.*, 2008. Advancing paternal age and bipolar disorder. *Archives of general psychiatry*, 65 (9), 1034.

Giddens, A., 1998. Risk society: the context of British politics. *In*: J. Franklin, ed. *The politics of risk society*. Malden, MA: Blackwell, 23–34.

Gross, S.E. and Shuval, J.T., 2008. On knowing and believing: prenatal genetic screening and resistance to 'risk-medicine'. *Health, risk & society*, 10 (6), 549–564.

Hallgrimsdottir, H.K., Benoit, C., and Phillips, R., 2013. The mother-citizen and the working girl: first-wave feminist citizenship claims in Canada and discursive opportunities for twenty-first century childcare policy. *Canadian review of sociology/revue canadienne de sociologie*, 50 (1), 27–51.

Hallgrimsdottir, H.K., Phillips, R., and Benoit, C., 2006. Fallen women and rescued girls: social stigma and media narratives of the sex industry in Victoria, BC, from 1980 to 2005*. *Canadian review of sociology/revue canadienne de sociologie*, 43 (3), 265–280.

Hanson, B., 2003. Questioning the construction of maternal age as a fertility problem. *Health care for women international*, 24 (3), 166–176.

Hays, S., 1996. *The cultural contradictions of motherhood*. New Haven, CT: Yale University Press.

Jahromi, B.N. and Husseini, Z., 2008. Pregnancy outcome at maternal age 40 and older. *Taiwanese journal of obstetrics and gynecology*, 47 (3), 318–321.

Jasen, P., 1997. Race, culture, and the colonization of childbirth in northern Canada. *Social history of medicine*, 10 (3), 383–400.

Koven, S. and Michel, S., 1990. Womanly duties: maternalist politics and the origins of welfare states in France, Germany, Great Britain, and the United States, 1880–1920. *The American historical review*, 95 (4), 1076–1108.

Lagerwey, M.D., 1999. Nursing, social contexts, and ideologies in the early United States birth control movement*. *Nursing inquiry*, 6 (4), 250–258.

Leavitt, J.W., 1987. The growth of medical authority: technology and morals in turn-of-the-century obstetrics. *Medical anthropology quarterly*, 1 (3), 230–255.

Lisonkova, S., *et al.*, 2011. Effect of older maternal age on birth outcomes in twin pregnancies: a population-based study. *Journal of perinatology*, 31 (2), 85–91.

Locke, A. and Budds, K., 2013. 'We thought if it's going to take two years then we need to start that now': age, infertility risk and the timing of pregnancy in older first-time mothers. *Health, risk & society*, 15, 525–542.

Loudon, I., 1992. *Death in childbirth: an international study of maternal care and maternal mortality 1800–1950*. Oxford: Clarendon Press.

Lupton, D., 2012. 'Precious cargo': foetal subjects, risk and reproductive citizenship. *Critical public health*, 22 (3), 329–340.

Lyon, D., 2001. *Surveillance society*. Buckingham: Open University Press.

Lyon, D., 2003. Surveillance technology and surveillance society. *In*: T.J. Misa, P. Brey, and A. Feenberg, eds. *Modernity and technology*. Cambridge, MA: MIT Press, 161.

Markens, S., Browner, C.H., and Mabel Preloran, H., 2010. Interrogating the dynamics between power, knowledge and pregnant bodies in amniocentesis decision making. *Sociology of health & illness*, 32 (1), 37–56.

McDonald, K., Amir, L., and Davey, M.-A., 2011. Maternal bodies and medicines: a commentary on risk and decision-making of pregnant and breastfeeding women and health professionals. *BMC public health*, 11 (Suppl. 5), S5.

McLaren, A., 1978. Birth Control and Abortion in Canada, 1870–1920. *Canadian historical review*, 59 (3), 319–340.

Morantz, R.M., 1977. Making women modern: middle class women and health reform in 19th century America. *Journal of social history*, 10 (4), 490–507.

OECD, 2012. *OECD family database*. Paris: OECD.

Perrier, M., 2013. No right time: the significance of reproductive timing for younger and older mothers' moralities. *The sociological review*, 61 (1), 69–87.

Pierce, J.B., 2008. Science, advocacy, and the sacred and intimate things of life: representing motherhood as a progressive era cause in women's magazines. *American periodicals: a journal of history, criticism, and bibliography*, 18 (1), 69–95.

Plant, R.J. and Van Der Klein, M., 2012. Introduction. *In*: M. Van Der Klein, eds. *Maternalism reconsidered: motherhood, welfare and social policy in the twentieth century*. New York: Berghahn Books, 1–21.

Richardson, E.H. and Turner, B.S., 2001. Sexual, intimate or reproductive citizenship? *Citizenship studies*, 5 (3), 329–338.

Richardson, T.R., 1989. *The century of the child: the mental hygiene movement and social policy in the United States and Canada*. Albany: State University of New York Press.

Riessman, C.K., 1983. Women and medicalization: a new perspective. *Social policy*, 14 (1), 3–18.

Root, R. and Browner, C.H., 2011. Cultural context of reproductive health. *In*: P. Van Look, K. Heggenhougen, and S.R. Quah, eds. *Sexual and reproductive health: a public health perspective*. Burlington, MA: Academic Press, 314–319.

Ruhl, L., 1999. Liberal governance and prenatal care: risk and regulation in pregnancy. *Economy and society*, 28 (1), 95–117.

Shaw, R.L. and Giles, D.C., 2009. Motherhood on ice? A media framing analysis of older mothers in the UK news. *Psychology & health*, 24 (2), 221–236.

Shelton, N. and Johnson, S., 2006. 'I think motherhood for me was a bit like a double-edged sword': the narratives of older mothers. *Journal of community & applied social psychology*, 16 (4), 316–330.

Shuttleworth, S., 1993/1994. A mother's place is in the wrong. *New scientist*, December/January, 38–40.

Silva, S. and Machado, H., 2010. Uncertainty, risks and ethics in unsuccessful in vitro fertilisation treatment cycles. *Health, risk & society*, 12 (6), 531–545.

Smajdor, A., 2009. Between fecklessness and selfishness: is there a biologically optimal time for motherhood? *In*: F. Simonstein, ed. *Reprogen-ethics and the future of gender*. New York: Springer, 105–117.

Smith-Rosenberg, C. and Rosenberg, C., 1973. The female animal: medical and biological views of woman and her role in nineteenth-century America. *The journal of American history*, 60 (2), 332–356.

Sutcliffe, A.G., *et al.*, 2012. The health and development of children born to older mothers in the United Kingdom: observational study using longitudinal cohort data. *British medical journal*, 345, 318.

Szreter, S., 2003. The population health approach in historical perspective. *American journal of public health*, 93 (3), 421–431.

Torrey, E.F., *et al.*, 2009. Paternal age as a risk factor for schizophrenia: how important is it? *Schizophrenia research*, 114 (1), 1–5.

Tucker, W.H., 1998. Keeping America sane: psychiatry and eugenics in the United States and Canada, 1880–1940. *Journal of the American Medical Association*, 279 (6), 477–478.

Valverde, M., 2008a. *The age of light, soap, and water: moral reform in English Canada, 1885–1925*. Toronto, ON: University of Toronto Press.

Valverde, M., 2008b. Racial purity, sexual purity, and immigration policy. *In*: W.B. Toronto, ed. *The history of immigration and Racism in Canada: essential readings*. Toronto, ON: Canadian Scholars' Press, 175–187.

Vézina, M. and Turcotte, M., 2009. Forty-year-old mothers of pre-school children: a profile. *In*: Statistics Canada, ed. *Canadian social trends*. Ottawa, ON: Statistics Canada.

Webster, A., 2002. Innovative health technologies and the social: redefining health, medicine and the body. *Current sociology*, 50 (3), 443–457.

Weir, L., 2006. *Pregnancy, risk, and biopolitics: on the threshold of the living subject*. New York: Routledge.

White, L.A., 2002. Ideas and the welfare state explaining child care policy development in Canada and the United States. *Comparative political studies*, 35 (6), 713–743.

Wrede, S., Benoit, C., and Einarsdottir, T., 2008. Equity and dignity in maternity care provision in Canada, Finland and Iceland. *The Canadian journal of public health*, 99, S16–S21.

Wrede, S., Benoit, C., and Einarsdottir, T., 2009. Equity and dignity in maternity care provision in Canada, Finland and Iceland. *The Canadian journal of public health*, 99, S16–S21.

'I don't think it's risky, but...': pregnant women's risk perceptions of maternal drinking and smoking

Raphaël Hammer and Sophie Inglin

University of Health Sciences (HESAV), Institute of Health Research, University of Applied Sciences and Arts, Western Switzerland (HES-SO), Lausanne, Switzerland

In Switzerland, official recommendations relating to alcohol and tobacco use during pregnancy are based on a zero-tolerance policy. However, epidemiological research indicates that some pregnant women do not adhere to the abstinence principle, and this raises the issue of how pregnant women identify and respond to health risks. This article draws on a sociocultural study of 50 mainly white, partnered and educated pregnant women carried out in Switzerland between May 2008 and June 2009. The study used semi-structured interviews that examined how and in what ways pregnancy had changed women's consumption of alcohol and tobacco and their perceptions of their riskiness. In this article we draw on these data to examine participants' perceptions of the risks of smoking and drinking during pregnancy. We examine three main issues: women's understandings of official recommendations, their contextualisation of risk in daily life and the moral issues which they saw surrounding smoking and drinking during pregnancy. We found that the women in our study perceived drinking and smoking during pregnancy as different types of risks with different meanings. The participants contextualised official recommendations about drinking during pregnancy and had their own views about its riskiness. In contrast all participants saw smoking as harmful and risky irrespective of the level of consumption. The pregnant women in our study saw smoking during pregnancy as a risk-taking behaviour and a failure to act in the best interest of the foetus. In contrast, under certain conditions, they saw moderate drinking of alcohol during pregnancy as acceptable and responsible behaviour.

Introduction

In the late twentieth century, public health experts have identified smoking and drinking during pregnancy as significant public health problems that are harmful to the developing foetus. Public health experts have linked heavy cigarette smoking during pregnancy to spontaneous abortions, low birth weights, premature births and sudden infant death syndromes, as well as adverse cognitive and behavioural outcomes in children (Shea and Steiner 2008) and they have linked heavy drinking during pregnancy to birth defects, neurodevelopmental disorders and childhood mental health problems (O'Leary and Bower 2012). However, there is less consensus amongst public health experts about the effects of a low or moderate level of smoking or drinking on the foetus (Huizink and Mulder 2006, Henderson *et al.* 2007). Although the evidence is not clear cut, most public health experts and policy experts have adopted a precautionary approach advocating complete abstinence from both smoking and drinking during pregnancy (Lowe and Lee 2010).

This approach is evident in Switzerland, where most of the key participants in health policy making, the Federal Office of Public Health, the Federation of Swiss Physicians and the Swiss Federation of Midwives recommend that pregnant women and women planning to become pregnant avoid all alcohol and tobacco consumption. This abstinence approach has informed recent information and awareness campaigns. Poster campaigns advocating no smoking during pregnancy started at the end of the 1990s, and the no-drinking campaigns started in 2003 based on the slogan 'no alcohol, baby on board'. As Lupton has noted, such campaigns are part of a broader development in which 'the pregnant woman is surrounded by a complex network of discourses and practices directed at the surveillance and regulation of her body' (1999, pp. 59–60).

However, in most Western countries, epidemiological research indicates that such campaigns have had limited impact and that many women do not stop smoking or drinking during pregnancy. For example in Switzerland, Keller *et al.* (2009) found that 13% of pregnant women reported that they were smoking while pregnant, and Meyer-Leu *et al.* (2011) found that 40% of pregnant women carried on drinking alcohol, of whom 8% said they drank moderately and only 1% heavily. There is some existing evidence that the way in which pregnant women assess risks is different to that of public health experts. For example Kesmodel and Kesmodel (2002) found that most pregnant women in their study did not consider drinking 'once in a while' as dangerous for their baby, and Grange *et al.* (2006) and Haslam and Draper (2001) found that pregnant smokers also tend to minimise the risk of their smoking to their baby. Such findings suggest that there is a difference between expert and pregnant women's views of risk, but it is not clear how and in what ways pregnant women respond to advice and if they see a difference between drinking and smoking. In this article we aim to contribute to an understanding of the relationship between health, risk and society by examining pregnant women's perceptions of the risks of smoking and drinking during pregnancy and exploring in what ways they perceive differences between the risks of these two forms of behaviour.

Perception of risk of drinking and smoking during pregnancy

In this article we take a sociocultural approach to risk towards examining the ways in which social processes influence individuals' perception of risk, and we consider the meaning which individuals give to risk. As Arnoldi (2009) has argued, in contrast to the psychological approach, which focuses on the role played by information and individuals' cognitive processes (Joffe 2003), the sociocultural approach is based on the assumption that variations in individuals' conceptualisations of and responses to risks are not prompted by intrinsic characteristics of the danger itself. Rather researchers using the sociocultural approach focus on the ways in which risk perceptions are shaped by the particular sociocultural settings in which individuals live (Wildavsky and Dake 1990). These researchers take the view that the ways people perceive and manage risks differ because they hold distinct beliefs, values and worldviews that are shaped by the various social and cultural contexts of their everyday lives. In this approach the level of scientific knowledge about risks is one of the numerous elements that influence lay perceptions of risk (Zinn 2008, Codern *et al.* 2010).

In the context of pregnancy, while pregnant women may be aware of health warnings about dangers of smoking and drinking, they are unlikely to be aware of the evidence and scientific reasoning that underpins such warnings (Haslam and Draper 2000, Guillemont *et al.* 2006, Codern *et al.* 2010). Thus how they respond to and interpret such warnings is likely to be affected by the context of their everyday lives.

However, as Arnoldi has noted, elucidating precisely 'how culture acts as a perceptual filter' (2009, p. 107) is at the core of a sociological understanding of differences in lay risk perception, as culture operates 'in very diffuse and indirect ways' (2009, p. 107). Uncovering the influence of culture on how people conceptualise and experience risk encompasses a wide range of contextual factors. How individuals make sense of risks pertains to various factors, such as political, institutional and legal considerations, as well as social norms, habits and socio-economic conditions. Regarding risk perception, therefore, empirical research has sought to examine the different aspects of cultural influences.

Douglas (1985) provides one possible starting point indicating that cultures are symbolic frameworks which individuals use to identify, make sense of and manage risks. Such symbolic frameworks have moral connotations, as the very notion of risk marks some behaviours as good and others as bad (Lupton, 2011). It is possible to identify some of the key elements of the symbolic framework of pregnancy in contemporary developed societies. Babies are highly valued, and pregnant women are expected to be 'good mothers' acting as a 'safe' repository for their babies by engaging in self-surveillance and following medical recommendations (Copelton 2007, Bessett 2010, Knaak 2010). Within this framework, drinking alcohol and smoking cigarettes are self-evidently hazardous and harmful to the baby, and women are expected to use their willpower to stop drinking and smoking when they become pregnant (Lupton 1999). Thus, in public health and broader societal discourses, maternal drinking and smoking are health-related risks, and pregnant women are required to be social responsible and exert self-control to avoid such behaviours (Oakley 1989, Armstrong 2003, Kukla 2010).

There is some research on the impact of public health policies on maternal smoking and drinking (Armstrong and Abel 2000, Oaks 2001, Drabble *et al.* 2011). For example Drabble *et al.* (2011) have examined the ways in which policies have shaped lay perceptions of drinking during pregnancy from one country to another. Helweg-Larsen *et al.* (2010) noted the difference between a 'smoking-prohibitive culture' (the United States) and a 'smoking-lenient culture' (Denmark) and considered the ways this influenced lay risk perception; Danish respondents were more likely to minimise their personal risks and held less moralised attitudes.

Some researchers (see Drabble *et al.* 2011) have also examined the ways in which collective beliefs and social practices, about smoking and drinking, have influenced perceptions of risk and patterns of consumption and have noted difference between smoking and drinking. In countries with 'tobacco denormalisation policies' (Bell *et al.* 2011, p. 7), smoking is increasingly stigmatised (Sei-Hill and Shanahan 2003, Godeau 2009). In contrast, alcohol policies have concentrated on responsible drinking (Bell *et al.* 2011), and in Western countries, drinking is seen as an individual lifestyle choice, rather than an unhealthy behaviour (Gaussot 2004). However, lay perceptions of smoking and drinking can also be affected by social categorisation: moderate and episodic maternal drinking seems to be more tolerated and perceived as less risky among women with higher levels of education in comparison with less-educated women (Audet *et al.* 2006, April *et al.* 2010, Toutain 2010).

While public health experts advice pregnant women to abstain from both smoking and drinking as part of the responsible behaviour of a 'good mother' who nurtures and protects her baby, it is not clear whether pregnant women see risk in the same way. While there have been some studies which explore perceptions of drinking or smoking, we are not aware of any studies that have examined and contrasted pregnant women's perception of both forms of behaviour. In this article we aim to fill this gap by exploring differences in how pregnant women perceive the risks related to alcohol and tobacco use in everyday life. We start by examining differences in women's attitudes towards the official recommendation of abstaining from alcohol and tobacco. We then examine the contextualised meanings of maternal drinking and smoking by exploring the circumstances in which women consider such behaviours to be acceptable and harmless. Finally, we examine the distinct forms of moralisation that apply to maternal smoking and drinking behaviours.

Data and methods

This article draws on data from a study of 50 pregnant women carried out in the French-speaking part of Switzerland between May 2008 and June 2009. This study used semi-structured interviews conducted to explore these women's experiences of pregnancy, attitudes towards the professional follow-up and information women receive, and the management of risks related to pregnancy (Manaï *et al.* 2010, Hammer and Burton-Jeangros 2013). To be eligible for the study, the participants had to have a normal pregnancy, thus excluding high-risk pregnancies and those exhibiting any pathology. We recruited participants through the social networks of the members of the research team, small posters in commercial centres, private obstetrician-gynaecologists' and mid-wives' offices and advertisements on web sites associated with family issues. These approaches were used in conjunction with snowball sampling.

The participants in our study were aged between 24 and 41 years. Most of them were interviewed between 16 and 28 weeks of pregnancy, and half of them were expecting their first child. All of the participants were living with a male partner, and most were married. Forty-one were Swiss citizens. Six participants were from other European countries, and three participants from countries outside Europe. While we did not ask the participants questions related to their income, all were in paid employment, with the exception of four women who were housewives and one who was a student. Thirty participants had university degrees (tertiary level), and 20 were classified at the secondary level. As our participants were overwhelmingly European, partnered and educated, our findings cannot be generalised to other groups of pregnant women. This is further discussed in the Discussion section.

The interviews asked participants about use of alcohol and tobacco and any changes in use since becoming pregnant, their views regarding dangerous and safe consumption during pregnancy, the information received from health professionals, their thoughts regarding official recommendations and attitudes towards other mothers' consumption. Raphaël Hammer and Samuele Cavalli each conducted almost half of the 50 interviews, and Claudine Burton-Jeangros conducted the remaining ones. The interviews lasted on average for 75 minutes and were transcribed verbatim and manually coded using Atlas.ti. A thematic analysis was performed on interview extracts related to knowledge, behaviours and attitudes regarding alcohol and tobacco consumption. All quotes from the interviews used in this study were translated from French into English. The Research Ethics Committee of the local medical association approved the study protocol.

Findings

Abstinence: compliance and questioning

All of the women in our study acknowledged that smoking or drinking during pregnancy were behaviours that might be harmful for the foetus, referring to the information provided by their attending obstetrician or midwife and to other sources such as public health campaigns, brochures and books or magazines for expectant mothers. While participants never challenged the hazardousness of drinking and smoking during pregnancy, their attitudes towards the official recommendation of abstinence were different and varied from compliance to questioning.

Most of the women in this study endorsed the abstinence principle, and when they became pregnant, they quit smoking or drinking alcohol, treating them in the same way. For example, Lucy[1] described her decision not to drink in terms of baby's well-being:

> I enjoy drinking a glass of wine but at this time I would say... for the baby, we'll go without it, that's it. I read complete abstinence is better.

Ex-smokers such as Melinda indicated that they had stopped before they became pregnant:

> So he [her obstetrician] asked me whether I used to smoke, well, I stopped a year ago (laughs) for prevention.

The participants who said that they abstained from smoking and drinking presented themselves as responsible mothers who avoided the risk of harming their baby. However, while women in this study tended to accept official advice that smoking was harmful, there was less agreement about drinking alcohol. Some of them questioned the need for total abstinence from drinking and suggested that occasional drinking could be safe.

Some participants argued that alcohol was different because experts differed over their advice about drinking. These women noted that official advice had changed from recommending moderation in drinking to total abstinence in pregnancy. Géraldine suggested that such changes indicated total abstinence was not based on solid evidence but was 'a fashion thing'. For Marie, there was a strong consensus that smoking was harmful that did not exist in relationship to drinking during pregnancy:

> I have the feeling that when it comes to cigarettes, it's much more clear in people's minds [that] it's bad... cigarettes are known to be harmful... whether you smoke one or two cigarettes... regarding alcohol... there truly are people who say and think that you definitely can drink a glass of wine while eating, even every day, and others who say 'oh how horrible, we should never drink a glass of alcohol while pregnant', so I really hear both points of view [about drinking].

For some women in our study the public health message was unclear. They were uncertain whether they should stop drinking all of the time or most of the time (Kesmodel and Kesmodel 2002, Raymond *et al.* 2009). For example, Valérie was unclear about what she was expected to do: 'Where is the limit of no alcohol? Is it zero alcohol or... well a little liqueur or....'.

Furthermore some participants referred to the flexible position about occasional moderate drinking they received from health professionals in antenatal sessions. For example Marie downplayed the official recommendation arguing that her midwife had been happy for her to have the occasional drink:

> I drink a little glass from time to time, and she [her midwife] told me 'it's OK' and that's it... so for her, it was acceptable.

Some of the women in the study drew on their own knowledge and experience of drinking to claim that moderate drinking was not harmful. Monica argued that moderate drinking in pregnancy was quite common and that there was no evidence it was harmful:

> Everyone drinks moderately while pregnant without anything happening, so I think [avoiding alcohol entirely while pregnant] is a bit extremist.

Similarly Françoise drew on her own observations of her friends and relatives claiming that:

> I have seen a lot of women who have been drinking a bit... not daily and they did not have horrific consequences.

For these women, personal experience was a more trustworthy source than science in shaping their judgements of risk. The scientific evidence did not seem relevant to their own experiences (Benn *et al.* 1999, Dunn 2004). For many women in our study, failure to comply with the abstinence principle on certain occasions did not involve taking irresponsible risks. Thus Eugénie, who had drunk alcohol during her previous pregnancies giving birth to two healthy children, claimed to be able to know 'what is right or wrong' and said she was drinking three glasses of wine or beer per week during her current pregnancy.

Contextualisation of risk in daily life

Drinking and smoking form part of everyday life, and in this section we explore the circumstances in which the women in our study felt it was not risky to smoke or drink. Regarding alcohol, the women in our study suggested that the type of alcohol, the quantity drunk and the frequency of drinking affected riskiness. In terms of type of alcohol the participants differentiated spirits from wine and beer. Drinking spirits was considered dangerous, while drinking wine was acceptable, as it involved little risk to the baby. For example, Françoise did not perceive drinking beer as a dangerous behaviour:

> I don't think that drinking a beer for a few months may compromise baby's health, honestly... but your doctor will never tell you that!

The women also stressed that to be safe, wine or beer had to be drunk occasionally and in moderation. For example, Margaret described her 'safe' drinking in the following way:

> Well, I still drink, that is a glass of red wine, but really... once every two weeks, something like that... I drink one beer once in a while, or even two, but not more than that.

Such drinking was assumed safe and acceptable because, as Laurence pointed out, she did not get drunk:

> I haven't got drunk since I got pregnant (laughs), but I drink a little glass from time to time or a beer without worries.

Some participants also insisted on avoiding risks by drinking slowly and referred to bodily signs as indicating a potential risk. For example, Adeline, who had 'no qualms when taking a sip [of wine]' talked about feeling pins and needles in the legs or head spinning as warning signals:

> This is what stopped me sometimes when I offered myself a glass and when I felt a bit of the drunk sensation.

As opposed to any sort of excessive consumption, such as being drunk or drinking regularly, which were associated with risk-taking, moderate alcohol use was considered a reasonable behaviour.

For several of the women in the study, 'drinking once in a while' was compatible with claims of abstinence, such as 'I don't drink alcohol' or 'I've given up alcohol'. As Noémie noted, these were exceptions to the general rule that she did not drink:

> During a good meal I drink wine, or for the aperitif I enjoy drinking a little glass. I sometimes drink half a glass to toast, such as when I celebrated my 30th birthday or on other occasions. I don't think it's risky, but otherwise it's true that I've given up alcohol.

The women in our study suggested that the exceptions to the general abstention rule occurred during social celebrations at which they were expected to participate by 'clinking glasses'. Such occasions legitimated drinking alcohol in certain Western societies as a vector of sociability and integration (Testa and Leonard 1995, Gaussot 2004). Women's accounts in our study were no exception to this cultural representation, as Elodie stated: 'it's part of our eating habits to drink a glass of wine during the meal'. Moreover, as reported by several women, drinking a glass of wine with a meal was not seen as risk-taking behaviour, while drinking alcohol on an empty stomach was perceived as a risky behaviour. Marie noted that: 'If I have already eaten well and I drink a little glass of red wine, I do not feel that I put my baby at risk'.

In contrast to drinking, the women in our study considered tobacco consumption during pregnancy to be dangerous irrespective of the amount consumed, the circumstances and means of consumption. Some did justify smoking but only as the lesser of two evils, that is the harm caused by continuing to smoke (including reducing the number of cigarettes) offset against the harm that might be caused if they stopped smoking. Some participants argued that quitting smoking abruptly was considered harmful for their baby because it reduced their capacity to cope with stress. Elodie argued that smoking was both pleasurable and the lesser of two evils:

> I still smoke, and I've chosen to smoke two cigarettes per day in the evening because I enjoy it and I assume it's better to smoke them than bang my head against the wall.

Most of the women in our study who carried on smoking indicated that they had sought and gained professional approval for their trade-off strategy. For example, Camille indicated that her obstetrician had set an upper limit for her smoking:

> He [obstetrician] told me that I could smoke up to five cigarettes, not more, and that I shouldn't get stressed out, that it shouldn't be a cause for anxiety.

The morality of maternal drinking and smoking

The women in our study placed drinking and smoking in a moral context and saw these behaviours in terms of dependency, self-control, personal responsibility, guilt and social control. Such moral evaluation was more evident in relationship to smoking than drinking.

The participants saw smoking during pregnancy as a moral issue characterised by the tension between dependency and self-control. The smokers in our study described smoking as an addiction and, both smokers and non-smokers used the term *drug* to emphasise the difficulty of controlling smoking behaviour. The smokers in our study all indicated that they struggled with their addiction and were trying to reduce the number of cigarettes they smoked but said they felt guilty that they could not stop completely. For example, Elodie described her struggle in the following way:

> I try hard but it's very difficult [to quit smoking], and I feel guilty saying to myself, well if I have a baby of two kilos instead of three, it will be my fault... even though no one could tell me with certainty, that's what I tell myself, but it doesn't work.

Even though the women in our study accepted the addictive nature of tobacco, they still felt pregnant women were responsible for controlling their own behaviour and not exposing their babies to the harmful effects of tobacco. For example Justine, an ex-smoker, stated that every pregnant woman should be able to put her baby first and give up smoking:

> As an ex-smoker I know how difficult it is to give it up, but at the same time I think that if this effort can't be made... I think that a pregnant woman should not smoke at all, really, even not one cigarette.

Participants felt that a pregnant woman who did not give up smoking had failed in her moral duty and had failed to use her willpower to overcome her addiction. Women in our study who carried on smoking felt guilty and felt that they had failed to be a good mother. Maryse described the moral tension between dependency and desire to comply with the abstinence principle in the following way:

> I really would like to give up completely. I actually did it two months ago. I had reduced to a third of cigarette. I was really proud of myself, but I have started smoking more cigarettes again, each time I have the feeling of guilt, that's clear... when I smoke, I would like it if she [the baby] kicked me to say 'oh that's no good', but she doesn't... that would help me a lot, because I know it's really not good.

Some of the women in our study felt that smoking during pregnancy was shocking. While some participants said they did not care if they saw a pregnant woman smoking in public, others considered it was disturbing or shocking. For example Melinda, an ex-smoker, stated that:

> I find it much more shocking to see a pregnant woman smoking, yet I have been a smoker... for me it is inconceivable to smoke while pregnant.

Some women found this behaviour so irresponsible that they felt obliged to intervene publicly to alter the behaviour of friends or relatives who smoke. For example, Delphine felt that the dangers of smoking during pregnancy were so obvious that she thought that if her friend knew the harm it caused she would not smoke. However, her husband persuaded her that it was her friend's private affair:

> I told myself, it's unbelievable, she doesn't know what she's doing to her baby, and when I wanted to tell her something, my husband told me 'shhh, it's not your business'.

Several of the women who smoked reported that their colleagues, friends or relatives had made critical comments or given them disapproving looks. Such moral pressure could be so strong that it resulted in 'shameful and secret smoking behaviour' (Guyon *et al.* 2007). For example, Laurence described how she concealed her smoking: 'I no longer dare to smoke out in the street, in public spaces, now that it [the pregnancy] is obvious'.

Drinking did not elicit the same opprobrium. When women in our study were critical about other pregnant women drinking, their criticism was directed at the quantity being drunk. They tended not to criticise occasional drinking. For example, Adeline differentiated between occasional drinking and drunkness:

> If I see [a pregnant woman] having a drink, I would tell myself that it could be me, but if I see her totally drunk, that's very different, I will tell myself, 'she's an idiot'.

For the women in our study, both smoking and drinking had a moral dimension, but these were differently expressed. Smoking was likely to be considered as a morally reprehensible feature of pregnant women's behaviours. In contrast, the women in our study framed drinking in moderation in terms of autonomy and personal responsibility and did not see occasional drinking as necessarily irresponsible or risky.

Discussion

In this article, we have added to the sociocultural literature on lay risk perception by examining the ways in which pregnant women compare and contrast the risks of smoking and drinking during pregnancy. Drawing on data from a study of overwhelmingly white, partnered and educated pregnant women in Switzerland, we have shown that participants did not perceive tobacco and alcohol use during pregnancy in the same way, each being framed by different meanings. We have highlighted major differences in these pregnant women's risk perception.

We found that the women in our study accepted public health recommendations that they should not smoke when they were pregnant as smoking was dangerous. Even the women who continued smoking while pregnant acknowledged that they should stop and when they were unable to do so negotiated a 'safe' level with health professionals. In contrast, the women in our study were more willing to question the abstinence message in relation to alcohol, arguing that there was no clear and agreed expert guidance and they had personal evidence that moderate drinking during pregnancy was safe. These findings are consistent with those of other studies (Kesmodel and Kesmodel 2002, Guillemont *et al.* 2006, Raymond *et al.* 2009).

Although the participants took the risk of smoking for granted, they did not necessarily perceive moderate drinking as dangerous. Most of them regarded maternal drinking as a potential risk but one which could be significantly reduced or eliminated by taking precautions, such as controlling the frequency and amount of drunk, not drinking spirits, drinking only in social settings such as meals or parties, drinking slowly and not drinking on an empty stomach. For these women, moderate drinking was reasonable and acceptable behaviour. Thus, most participants constructed their own representations of the riskiness of alcohol use during pregnancy.

Whatever their perceptions of the risks of maternal smoking and drinking, all the women in the study stated that the safety and well-being of their baby were their top priority and accepted that it was their responsibility to ensure a successful outcome of their pregnancy, the birth of a healthy baby (Lupton 2011). However, we found that drinking was less of a moral issue than smoking. The women in our study, including smokers, readily framed tobacco use in terms of failure to control oneself or to be a 'good mother' (Bessett 2010). In contrast, they saw 'drinking once in a while' as being compatible with being a responsible person who looked after herself and her baby. Their accounts regarding moderate alcohol consumption tended to be framed by notions of autonomy, whereas any tobacco use was viewed from the perspective of restraint or addiction. These findings indicate that the sense of being able to control risks and choose which ones to take constitutes an important feature shaping moralisation and lay perceptions of risks (Järvinen 2012). Our findings are consistent with the view that in contemporary developed societies, the emphasis on self-control and individual responsibility tends to deflect attention from the fact that 'bad choices' are shaped by factors beyond an individual's control, cultural pressures (Wikler 2002) and environmental factors (Callahan *et al.* 2000). Such a notion of responsibility cannot be absolute in a context in which individuals have different levels of control over their behaviours, which are influenced by social factors (Hiscock *et al.* 2011, Skagerström *et al.* 2011).

In this article, we argue that the contrasting cultural beliefs and practices related to alcohol and tobacco play a significant role in generating our participants' contrasting attitudes towards official recommendations, contextualisation of risk in daily life and moralisation. In Switzerland as in other countries, cultural beliefs and practices regarding alcohol and tobacco consumption are different (Bell *et al.* 2011).

On the legislative and political levels, tobacco has been subjected to significant restrictions in Switzerland.[2] Second-hand smoke and its effects on health have provoked lively public debates over the last few years and have been extensively covered in the Swiss mass media. A new law on second-hand smoke, which was enacted in May 2010, prohibits the use of tobacco in enclosed public spaces. More generally, tobacco consumption is clearly perceived to be dangerous, and second-hand smoke has evolved from being understood as a public nuisance to being understood as a toxin (Godeau 2009). This evolution towards an unfavourable social climate for smoking is observed in other countries such as the United States (Sei-Hill and Shanahan 2003). To a large extent, our data resonate with studies showing that maternal smoking is considered a shameful behaviour and is associated with social stigma (Guyon *et al.* 2007): pregnant smokers in our study expressed feelings of guilt, reported having experienced social control and some felt such substantial moral pressure that they gave up smoking in public spaces.

In Switzerland, alcohol enjoys fairly broad social acceptance as a part of the everyday life and social interactions. As in other Western countries, the social construct of 'good drinking' associates moderate drinking with a form of pleasure and identifies this activity as a component of sociability. Drinking wine is seen as an important part of such activities (Testa and Leonard 1995, Gaussot 2004). In our study, several participants readily framed drinking wine during meals, as well as 'clinking glasses' in celebrations of social events, as lifestyle elements. Moreover, the women in our study made a sharp distinction between moderate consumption of wine and beer, which they perceived to be safe, as opposed to drinking spirits, which they categorised as dangerous. This distinction reflects the pattern of alcohol consumption in Switzerland, where wine and beer are the most popular alcoholic beverages (Federal Office of Public Health 2012). In addition, while moderate alcohol consumption has some legitimacy and is perceived as having some health benefits, 'the idea of moderate consumption is almost entirely missing from contemporary discourses on tobacco' (Bell *et al.* 2011, p. 6).

In relationship to moral issues such as responsibility and self-control, our findings show that smoking during pregnancy was generally categorised as a personal failure and tended to be associated with notions of ill health and deviance (Sei-Hill and Shanahan 2003, Godeau 2009, Bell *et al.* 2011). In contrast, our findings show that the issue of moderate maternal drinking was frequently embedded in accounts referring to drinking in general as a social and cultural practice rather than a health issue (Gaussot 2004). In contrast, no woman in our study made references to cultural habits or social practices when discussing smoking during pregnancy. Our findings, therefore, suggest that cultural beliefs and practices surrounding smoking and drinking shape, to some extent, pregnant women's attitudes towards alcohol and tobacco.

Nevertheless, cultural beliefs and practices related to health matters are liable to change depending on various factors, such as public health messages and the attitudes of healthcare professionals. It should be noted that educational approaches have not consistently been effective and are difficult to evaluate because of time lags (Foxcroft *et al.* 2003). However, it is possible that, as a result of awareness campaigns on the risks of alcohol use during pregnancy, Swiss attitudes on alcohol may become less lenient in the future, as has been the case in other European countries. For example, a study conducted in France has shown that the introduction of a pictogram or sentence on alcoholic beverage bottles conveying the harmful effects – even in small doses – of alcohol during pregnancy can have a positive impact, insofar as the social norm on maternal drinking has moved towards 'zero alcohol' (Guillemont and Léon 2008).

Our study has a number of limitations. Given the overrepresentation of well-educated women in this sample, our findings cannot be generalised to other class backgrounds, in particular to pregnant women from disadvantaged backgrounds. Indeed, maternal drinking and smoking have been shown to vary according to socioeconomic status. Women from the highest socioeconomic sections of the population are more likely to consume alcohol during pregnancy (Copelton 2003), whereas those from lower socioeconomic sections are more likely to smoke when pregnant (Cnattingius 2004). Furthermore, the higher a pregnant woman's education level, the less likely she is to consider 'drinking once in a while' to be a risk for her baby (April *et al.* 2010, Toutain 2010), whereas those with less education consider alcohol use to be unacceptable whatever the quantity (Audet *et al.* 2006). Lastly, it must be emphasised that alcohol and tobacco use may have emotional benefits and operate as a means of coping with difficulties in daily life (Graham 1994, Haslam and Draper 2001). Depending on the context of their everyday lives, pregnant women may not necessarily perceive tobacco or alcohol use as paramount risks. Consequently, further studies could complement our findings by focussing on less well-educated pregnant women's perceptions of maternal smoking and drinking. Our findings cannot be generalised to other cultural contexts because, as noted above, each society has its own public health policy and cultural beliefs and practices regarding alcohol and tobacco, although there may be similarities between countries (Helweg-Larsen *et al.* 2010, Drabble *et al.* 2011).

Conclusion

In this article, we drew on data from a Swiss study of pregnant women to explore their assessments of risk during pregnancy and this enabled us to examine similarities and differences between the perceived risks of smoking and drinking during pregnancy. We found that these women's assessments of risks were shaped by contrasting meanings they ascribed to these two types of behaviour. They perceived smoking during pregnancy as a risk-taking behaviour involving the failure to act in the best interest of the baby. In contrast, under certain conditions, they saw moderate drinking during pregnancy as an acceptable and responsible behaviour. Overall, the participants viewed alcohol consumption during pregnancy as a minor issue compared to tobacco use. We have argued that differences in cultural beliefs and practices surrounding alcohol and tobacco in Switzerland may, to some extent, account for the different meanings that pregnant women in our study attributed to maternal drinking and smoking as health risks. Nevertheless, to fully understand the dynamics of risk perception in everyday life on these issues, further research is necessary to explore the complex relationships between cultural beliefs, social practices, public health policies and health professionals' information strategies and should involve pregnant women from various socioeconomic backgrounds.

Funding

This research was funded by a grant from the Swiss National Science Foundation.

Notes

1. All interviewees are referred to using pseudonyms.
2. http://www.bag.admin.ch/themen/drogen/00041/07322/07324/index.html?lang=fr.

References

April, N., et al., 2010. Représentations sociales et consommation d'alcool pendant la grossesse. *Drogues, santé et société*, 9 (2), 17–48.

Armstrong, E.M., 2003. *Conceiving risk, bearing responsibility, Fetal alcohol syndrome and the diagnosis of moral disorder*. Baltimore, MD: John Hopkins University Press.

Armstrong, E. and Abel, E., 2000. Fetal alcohol syndrome: the origins of a moral panic. *Alcohol and alcoholism*, 35 (3), 276–282.

Arnoldi, J., 2009. *Risk*. London: Polity Press.

Audet, C., et al., 2006. *Représentations de la consommation d'alcool pendant la grossesse et perceptions des messages de prévention chez des femmes enceintes*. Québec: Institut national de la santé publique du Québec.

Bell, K., McNaughton, D., and Salmon, A., ed., 2011. *Alcohol, tobacco and obesity. morality, mortality and the new public health*. London: Routledge.

Benn, C., Budge, R.C., and White, G.E., 1999. Women planning and experiencing pregnancy and childbirth: information needs and sources. *Nursing praxis in new zealand inc*, 14, 4–15.

Bessett, D., 2010. Negotiating normalization: the perils of producing pregnancy symptoms in prenatal care. *Social science & medicine*, 71 (2), 370–377.

Callahan, D., Koenig, B., and Minkler, M., 2000. Promoting health and preventing disease: ethical demands and social challenges. *In*: D. Callahan, ed. *Promoting healthy behavior*. Washington, DC: Georgetown University Press, 153–170.

Cnattingius, S., 2004. The epidemiology of smoking during pregnancy: smoking prevalence, maternal characteristics, and pregnancy outcomes. *Nicotine and tobacco research*, 6 (2), 125–140.

Codern, N., *et al.*, 2010. Risk perception among smokers: a qualitative study. *Risk analysis*, 30 (10), 1563–1571.

Copelton, D.A., 2003. *Pregnancy by the book: women's accomodation and resistance to medicalized pregnancy practices.* State University of New York: Binghampton University.

Copelton, D.A., 2007. 'You are what you eat': nutritional norms, maternal deviance, and neutralization of women's prenatal diets. *Deviant behavior*, 28 (5), 467–494.

Douglas, M., 1985. *Risk acceptability according to the social sciences.* New York: Russell Sage Foundation.

Drabble, L.A., *et al.*, 2011. Conceiving risk, divergent responses: perspectives on the construction of risk of FASD in six countries. *Substance use & misuse*, 46, 943–958.

Dunn, C., 2004. Lay advice on alcohol and tobacco during pregnancy. *Health care for women international*, 25 (1), 55–75.

[Federal Office of Public Health], 2012. *Monitorage suisse des addictions: Alcool.* Berne: Office fédéral de la santé publique.

Foxcroft, D.R., *et al.*, 2003. Longer-term primary prevention for alcohol misuse in young people: a systematic review. *Addiction*, 98 (4), 397–411.

Gaussot, L., 2004. *Modération et sobriété. Etudes sur les usages sociaux de l'alcool.* Paris: L'Harmattan.

Godeau, E., 2009. Comment le tabac est-il devenu une drogue? *Vingtième siècle. Revue d'histoire*, 102, 105–115.

Graham, H., 1994. Gender and class as dimensions of smoking behaviour in Britain: insights from a survey of mothers. *Social science & medicine*, 38 (5), 691–698.

Grange, G., *et al.*, 2006. Risk perception related to smoking among pregnant women. *Alcoologie et addictologie*, 28, 22S–25S.

Guillemont, J. and Léon, C., 2008. Alcool et grossesse: connaissances du grand public en 2007 et évolutions en trois ans. *Evolutions*, 15, 1–6.

Guillemont, J., *et al.*, 2006. Connaissances des Français sur les risques liés à la consommation d'alcool pendant la grossesse. *Evolutions*, 3, 1–4.

Guillemont, J. and Léon, C., 2008. Alcool et grossesse: connaissances du grand public en 2007 et évolutions en trois ans. *Evolutions*, 15, 1–6.

Guyon, L., *et al.*, 2007. Tabagisme et grossesse. Représentations sociales chez des mères québecoises. *Drogues, santé et société*, 6 (1), 105–142.

Hammer, R. and Burton-Jeangros, C., 2013. Tensions around risks in pregnancy: a typology of women's experiences of surveillance medicine. *Social science & medicine*, 93, 55–63.

Haslam, C. and Draper, E., 2000. Stage of change is associated with assessment of the health risks of maternal smoking among pregnant women. *Social science & medicine*, 51 (1), 1189–1196.

Haslam, C. and Draper, E., 2001. A qualitative study of smoking during pregnancy. *Psychology, health and medicine*, 6 (1), 95–99.

Helweg-Larsen, M., Tobias, M.R., and Cerban, B.M., 2010. Risk perception and moralization among smokers in the U.S. and Denmark: a qualitative approach. *British journal of health psychology*, 15, 871–886.

Henderson, J., Gray, R., and Brocklehurst, P., 2007. Systematic review of effects of low–moderate prenatal alcohol exposure on pregnancy outcome. *BJOG an international journal of obstetrics and gynaecology*, 114 (3), 243–252.

Hiscock, R., Judge, K., and Bauld, L., 2011. Social inequalities in quitting smoking: what factors mediate the relationship between socioeconomic position and smoking cessation? *Journal of Public Health*, 33 (1), 39–47.

Huizink, A.C. and Mulder, E.J., 2006. Maternal smoking, drinking or cannabis use during pregnancy and neurobehavioral and cognitive functioning in human offspring. *Neuroscience & biobehavioral reviews*, 30 (1), 24–41.

Järvinen, M., 2012. A will to health?: drinking, risk and social class. *Health, risk & society*, 14 (3), 241–256.

Joffe, H., 2003. Risk: from perception to social representation. *British journal of social psychology*, 42, 55–73.

Keller, R., *et al.*, 2009. *Tabagisme et grossesse: monitorage sur le tabac – Enquête suisse sur le tabagisme.* Zürich: Psychologisches Institut der Universität Zürich, Sozial- und Geshundeitpsychologie.

Kesmodel, U. and Kesmodel, P.S., 2002. Drinking during pregnancy: attitudes and knowledge among pregnant Danish women, 1998. *Alcoholism: clinical and experimental research*, 26 (10), 1553–1560.

Knaak, S., 2010. Contextualising risk, constructing choice: breastfeeding and good mothering in risk society. *Health, risk & society*, 12 (4), 345–355.

Kukla, R., 2010. The ethics and cultural politics of reproductive risk warnings: a case study of California's Proposition 65. *Health, risk & society*, 12 (4), 323–334.

Lowe, P.K. and Lee, E.J., 2010. Advocating alcohol abstinence to pregnant women: some observations about British policy. *Health, risk & society*, 12 (4), 301–311.

Lupton, D., 1999. Risk and the ontology of pregnant embodiment. *In*: D. Lupton, ed. *Risk and sociocultural theory*. Cambridge: Cambridge University Press, 59–85.

Lupton, D., 2011. The best thing for the baby': mothers' concepts and experiences related to promoting their infants' health and development. *Health, risk & society*, 13 (7–8), 637–651.

Manaï, D., Burton-Jeangros, C., and Elger, B., 2010. *Risques et informations dans le suivi de la grossesse: droit, éthique et pratiques sociales*. Bern: Stämpfli/Bruylant.

Meyer-Leu, Y., *et al.*, 2011. Association of moderate alcohol use and binge drinking during pregnancy with neonatal health. *Alcoholism: clinical and experimental research*, 35 (9), 1669–1677.

Oakley, A., 1989. Smoking in pregnancy: smokescreen or risk factor? Towards a materialist analysis. *Sociology of health & illness*, 11 (4), 311–334.

Oaks, L., 2001. *Smoking and Pregnancy: the politics of fetal protection*. New Brunswick, NJ: Rutgers University Press.

O'Leary, C. and Bower, C., 2012. Guidelines for pregnancy: what's an acceptable risk, and how is the evidence (finally) shaping up? *Drug and alcohol review*, 31 (2), 170–183.

Raymond, N., *et al.*, 2009. Pregnant women's attitudes towards alcohol consumption. *BMC public health*, 9 (175), 1–8.

Sei-Hill, K. and Shanahan, J., 2003. Stigmatizing smokers: public sentiment toward cigarette smoking and its relationship to smoking behaviors. *Journal of health communication: international perspectives*, 8 (4), 343–367.

Shea, A. and Steiner, M., 2008. Cigarette smoking during pregnancy. *Nicotine & tobacco research*, 10 (2), 267–278.

Skagerström, J., Chang, G., and Nilsen, P., 2011. Predictors of drinking during pregnancy: a systematic review. *Journal of women's health*, 20 (6), 901–913.

Testa, M. and Leonard, K.E., 1995. Social influences on drinking during pregnancy. *Psychology of addictive behaviors*, 9 (4), 258–268.

Toutain, S., 2010. What women in France say about alcohol abstinence during pregnancy. *Drug and acohol review*, 29, 184–188.

Wikler, D., 2002. Personal and social responsibility for health. *Ethics and international affairs*, 16, 47–55.

Wildavsky, A. and Dake, K., 1990. Theories of risk perception: who fears what and why? *American academy of arts and sciences*, 119 (4), 41–60.

Zinn, J.O., 2008. Heading into the unknown: everyday strategies for managing risk and uncertainty. *Health, risk & society*, 10 (5), 439–450.

The risk of being 'too honest': drug use, stigma and pregnancy

Camille Stengel[a,b]

[a]School for Social Policy, Sociology and Social Research, University of Kent, Canterbury, UK;
[b]School of Criminology, Faculty of Law, Eötvös Loránd University, Budapest, Hungary

In this article, I examine the ways in which risk is constructed and managed by those involved in the pregnancy and childbirth of women who use drugs, including the women themselves. I discuss how constructions of risk influence maternal care outcomes and the understanding of choice, often in the form of stigmatisation. In this article, I draw on data from a qualitative research study that I conducted in 2011 in a western Canada city in which I interviewed 13 pregnant and parenting women who had used drugs during their pregnancy. In this article, I show how the everyday risk construction of pregnancy, labour and delivery is compounded significantly by drug use and the stigmatisation associated with this perceived risk-taking behaviour. The participants in the study often internalised this understanding of risk and this manifested itself in delays in accessing maternal health and social care services. The women in the study had different understandings of risk and these were structured by the women's own understanding of general risk factors during their pregnancy, as well as their experiences of the constructions of risk and risk management by health and social care professionals. While structural life chances can constrain women's feelings of self-efficacy, services that promote clients' ability to make choices can facilitate reduced stigmatisation and facilitate the development of more compassionate and autonomous approaches to risk management.

Introduction

In this article, I examine the ways in which risk is constructed and managed by those involved in the pregnancy and childbirth of women who use drugs, including the women themselves. Drug use in this context refers to both illicit drugs and licit drugs (opioids, benzodiazepines, amphetamines, alcohol and tobacco), whose consumption during pregnancy is commonly categorised as risk-taking behaviour. I discuss how constructions of risk, often in the form of stigmatisation, influence maternal care outcomes and understanding of choice. Framed against a discussion of relevant literature surrounding risk categorisation of pregnant women who use drugs, I draw on data from original qualitative research conducted with women about their maternity care experiences in Canada. I use these data to examine how pregnant women understood the risks of taking drugs and how their understanding varied both in terms of their understanding of general risk factors during their pregnancy, as well as how their experiences of the ways in which health and social care professionals constructed and managed risk.

I start this article with a discussion of the relevant literature on risk, pregnancy, drug use and stigma. I then outline the methodology of the research study of women in western

Canada who used drugs during pregnancy that generated the data that I draw on in this article. I discuss three main factors which shape these women's experiences of risk categorisation and management: their interaction with health and social care professionals; their response to advice and guidance from the Ministry of Child and Family Development; and their categorisation of the risks of drug use, especially their sense of this as stigmatised behaviour.

Pregnancy, risk and drug use

Pregnancy as risk

Feminist commentary have identified the ways in which the female body is a figurative symbol of fluidity and dynamic instability, which becomes literal when pregnant women are perceived as potentially dangerous vessels for their foetus (Butler 1990, Young 1994, Ettorre 2004, Lupton 2012). Pregnant bodies, and the event of pregnancy, labour and delivery have become constituted as potential sites for risk, and 'a pathology of pregnancy' pervades approaches to pregnant women in order to monitor this ambiguous status (Burton-Jeangros 2011). The dominant response of medical professionals is to seek to minimise and manage risk. This risk management is enacted through formal and informal actions and protocol through health and social professionals' interactions with pregnant women, as well as women's internalisation of social norms associated with risk. This lead to individualisation, that locates risk within the individual woman's body and is based on the assumption that women have the ability, and thus the responsibility, to manage potential risks in their lives during pregnancy and birth (Beck 1992). This understanding of risk as self-determined underpins the idea of pregnant women's self-efficacy, but also involves the allocation of personal blame when pregnant women fail to minimise risk, especially when they engage in 'risk behaviours' such as drug use. Salmon (2011) identifies this individualisation as 'reproductive citizenship', which connotes pregnant women as having a 'duty' to self-regulate their potentiality for risk, especially and primarily if the risk has potential to negatively affect the foetus. The concept of reproductive citizenship is based on utilising women's agency to make decisions about pregnancy-related risk founded on their own understandings of their body and their needs as autonomous individuals. Reproductive citizenship can be manifested as the socially constructed gender norms and expectations of the archetypal 'good mother'. Women who break these norms, especially during pregnancy, are labelled as additionally 'risky', and are subject to increased monitoring and control through formal and informal interventions (Campbell and Ettorre 2011).

Drug use as added risk

Drug use is often viewed as a deviant and self-destructive behaviour that is divorced from cultural norms, and is laden with moral judgments associated with 'choice' (Humphries 1999, Greaves and Poole 2008). Such attitudes are intensified through negative connotations and stigmatising assumptions about pregnant women who use drugs (Rutman et al. 2000, Radcliffe 2011). To be a pregnant woman who uses drugs is to deviate completely from gendered societal norms, and hence breaks down the basic structure of gendered relations that are dictated by rigid adherence to the notion of 'femininity' (Young 1994). Punitive policy responses and stigmatising attitudes to pregnant women who use drugs are an attempt to control this perceived 'breakdown of social order' and an idealistic effort to 'maintain social boundaries and divisions' (Tulloch and Lupton 2003, p. 7). Drug use, especially by women who are pregnant, provokes a double stigma towards women failing gendered expectations of femininity and motherhood (Boyd 2001, Pinkham and Malinowska-Sempruch 2007). In effect, women in this position are labelled as a twofold risk to society.

Risk manifested in stigma

Pregnant women who use drugs are subject to the powerful force of stigmatisation. Goffman (1963) a key theorist defined stigma as 'an attribute that links a person to an undesirable stereotype, leading other people to reduce the bearer from a whole and usual person to a tainted, discounted one' (p. 11). Goffman argued that being identified as having a moral 'failings' such as using drugs while pregnant resulted in an individual being ascribed a 'spoiled identity'. Through the medicalisation of pregnancy, and drug use as symptomatic of risk identification, this form of surveillance has served to stigmatise women and construct their behaviour as putative cause for anything that could go wrong during and after the pregnancy (Woolgar and Pawluch 1985). This can be seen in the media scare of 'crack babies' in the 1990s in the USA, and continues to be a justification for removing a child from their mothers' care. Stigma, judgement and discrimination are justified in terms of poor health outcomes for drug taking women but there is no evidence that they are effective in reducing the frequency of the undesirable behaviour such as drug use (Stubber and Myer 2008). Furthermore, adverse health outcomes may be linked to structural issues like inadequate food security, intimate partner violence or poverty, which are also factors in drug taking during pregnancy.

Campbell explains how 'gender failure – the social or psychological incapacity to perform within the constraints of normative femininity' can further add to the vilification a woman when she fails to conform to the gendered norms and heightened femininity expected due to pregnancy (2000, p. 154). Such stereotypes often typify pregnant women who use drugs as 'unfit mothers, out of control, and a danger to their children' (Boyd 1999). Such constructions of risk often become internalised by women, and assign total responsibility to the individual for their actions without taking into account context-specific and structural considerations.

Stigmatised women drug users have little or no control to resist or attempt to reverse the stigmatisation process on a structural level. Link and Phelan (2001) argue that stigmatisation has a large impact on an individual's life chances, and subsequently results in poor health behavioural outcomes. Fear of acquiring a stigmatising label often leads 'individuals to delay or avoid seeking treatment altogether, while those already labelled may decide to distance themselves from the label, forgoing treatment or becoming noncompliant' (Link and Phelan 2006, p. 528). Many research studies have found that internalised negative feelings of existing stereotypes about this vulnerable population are a common barrier for women accessing care services (Poole and Isaac 2001, Leslie and DeMarchi 2004, Macrory and Boyd 2007, Benoit et al. 2010, Campbell and Ettorre 2011). Fear of child removal as a result of societal stigmatisation is a factor in low uptake and retention rates of health and social services of pregnant women who use drugs (Davis and Yonkers 2012). Women are often afraid of being incarcerated or having their children taken from them, hence often do not seek out treatment options (Marcellus 2004, Friedman et al. 2009).

Thus to design health and social programmes that effectively recruit and deliver services to the target population, it is critical that the population themselves are the ones who are asked and talk about their needs. In this article, I address this issue by drawing on data from a research study in which I interviewed women who used drugs during pregnancy. The interviews were designed in part to engage with their experiences as the basis for designing a social and health care centre in the local community that will support women in similar life circumstances (the HerWay Home Programme).

Methodology

This article draws on some of the data from a larger, multi-level project[1] conducted on health and social services for women that was used to inform the development and delivery of the HerWay Home Programme. The Programme is collaborative maternity project that provides community-based care programme in the province of British Columbia. It is designed to offer a comprehensive range of support and services at a single access point, for pregnant women and new mothers (Davoren and Poag 2010). The services provided by the Programme aim to address the significant life challenges their clients face, including drug use, unstable housing and other adverse health outcomes.

The interviews that inform this article were carried out to assist with designing Programme in the pre-implementation phase. While it relatively common to undertake inter-view-based studies to evaluate programmes after they have opened (Uziel-Miller and Lyons 2000, Sword *et al.* 2004, Marshall *et al.* 2005), it is less common to use interview studies to identified aspects and services and strengthen the strategic planning of services before the intervention programme starts. The method of semi-structured interviews provided space for participants to articulate their experiences of risk identification and management during their pregnancy. For this research study I wanted to gain insight into how women who used drugs during pregnancy understood, responded and negotiated construction of risks with their health and social care provides, as well as within themselves.

I conducted the fieldwork during the first four months of 2011 in a city in western Canada.[2] The recruitment process began with three key individuals that were part of the network of organisations involved in developing the HerWay Home Programme, and was already providing services for pregnant women. These key individuals identified 10 suitable women who agreed to take part in the interviews and these women in turn identified a further three suitable participants. The criteria for recruiting participants were based on women who were dealing with issues of drug use during their pregnancy. The time length between their pregnancy and the interview was not relevant, as the purpose of the interviews were to capture women's experiences of using drugs while pregnant. The women were informed before the interview began that they could withdraw from the study at any time during and after the interview and to protect their identity all names used in this article are pseudonyms. None of the participants requested to withdraw from the study. The University of Victoria and the Vancouver Island Health Authority ethics committees approved the research proposal and design of this project.

The interviews

The interviews were designed to explore women's experiences of the pregnancy and birth (see Figure 1) and the sorts of facilities and service that they felt a new Programme should provide. While the issues of drug use and risk were not lead or explicit questions, the participants were given time and space to talk about their experiences and, as they had all used some form of drug during their pregnancy, issues of drug use, risk and responsibility were topics which they raised and discussed throughout the interviews.

HERWAY HOME PROGRAM: INDIVIDUAL INTERVIEW QUESTIONNAIRE

The following questions are about your life, health, pregnancy and birth experiences.
If you do not feel comfortable with a question you do not have to answer, and if you
like we can either skip the question or write the answer down on a piece of paper and put it in an envelope for me to read later. All of your responses remain confidential and anonymous. Do you have any questions before we begin?

Pregnancy
Q1. Please tell me about how you found out when you were pregnant.

Birthing experience
Q2. Please tell me about your experience with giving birth.

Your Health
Q3. What kinds of things are affecting your health and well being these days?

Your Children's Health
Q4. Is your child/children's health? How's their sleeping pattern, mood, eating habits?

HerWay Home Program

HerWay Home is an acronym for
Housing first,
Empowering,
Respect,
Woman,
Acceptance,
Your choice,
Health,
Opportunity,
Mothering and
Equality

Q5. What services do you think should be at the HerWay Home Program?

Anything Else?

Q6. Is there anything else you would like to talk about that hasn't been mentioned, or talk about something else in more detail?

Q7. Are you interested in potentially being part of the Women's Advisory Committee?

***THIS IS THE END OF THE INTERVIEW. THANK YOU FOR YOUR TIME!!**

Figure 1. Interview guide.

Before each interview began, I told the participants that the questions were meant to be a guide for conversation, and that ultimately *her* story and *her* experiences were the most important piece of information. This acknowledgement was meant to communicate to participants that *they* were the experts, and that they should not feel restrained by having to answer every question 'correctly'.

The interviews took on average between 45 and 60 minutes, with the shortest interview being just under a half hour, and the longest interview just over an hour and a half. In the interviews women provided accounts of their pregnancy and childbirth including their use of drugs. At the time of the interviews 11 women had given birth and the remaining two were still pregnant, one seven weeks into her pregnancy and the other six months. The average age range of participants was in the early twenties, with the youngest participant being 17 years old and the oldest participant recently turned 40 years old. The ages of their children ranged from five weeks to nine years old, and of them, seven had other children. Six women had other children prior to the pregnancy they discussed in the interviews. The women I interviewed identified using a range of substances, including heroin, methadone and other prescription drugs, crack and powder cocaine, crystal methamphetamine (meth), gamma hydroxybutanoic acid (GHB), marijuana, alcohol and tobacco. The majority of the participants stated that they were using more than one of these substances, especially alcohol and tobacco in conjunction with illicit drugs.

There were no questions about the women's race, ethnicity or citizenship during the interviews. Only one participant mentioned her ethnicity by identifying that she had a Native Status Card, an official government form of identification for people of a First Nations heritage. The other participants did not disclose any information about their ethnic, racial or cultural background. In the initial drafting stages the interview schedule consisted of both a demographic questionnaire and a series of semi-structured interview questions. Following debate amongst the research team it was decided not to include demographic data in the interview schedule due to fear that both a questionnaire and an interview may result in participant fatigue. In retrospect, this kind of data would have been helpful in order to gain a better understanding of the participants' socioeconomic status, age, level of completed education, ethnicity or race, cultural background, employment status, or other demographic factors beyond what they chose to reveal during the interviews. However, most of the participants mentioned their age at some point during the interview, and described situations surrounding their low socioeconomic status.

Another limitation of this study is the narrow scope of the sample. While utilising key informants already involved with HerWay Home Programme assisted with a speedy recruitment response, it also resulted in a lack of diversity from participants who had received similar care from these gatekeeper organisations, and possibly even from the same care providers. This study should therefore be read as exploratory and there may be additional issues worth exploring for further research, as mentioned in the previous section.

Analysis

I used an inductive thematic approach to analysis, which derived from a constructivist approach grounded theory, in which theory is developed from the research (Glaser and Strauss 1967). Grounded theory from a constructivist strategy involves 'flexible, heuristic strategies' of qualitative research that differ from the positivist origins of ground theory, and is based in an understanding of various forms of knowledge that is co-created by both the researcher and those who are the subject of research (Charmaz 2008, p. 250). Using grounded theory as a method of analysis involves including various stages of coding, constant comparative techniques and open coding (Glaser and Strauss 1967, Charmaz and Mitchell 2001). I organised the data 'into a logical, systematic, and explanatory scheme' in order to develop thematic categories that could be organised into the findings of the research (Collingridge and Gantt 2008, p. 393). However, unlike grounded theory, I did not continue collecting data until I reached the point of theoretical saturation, the point at which no new categories were being identified (Glaser and Strauss 1967, Charmaz and Mitchell 2001). As a result, the data analysis followed more general research strategies that involved bracketing sections of data from the transcriptions, conducting initial and secondary coding, and completing subsequent waves of thematic groupings of the emerging codes.

I started analysis soon after each interview ended; writing down initial thoughts and notes in a research journal as soon as was possible. Some of these thoughts were later shared with a research assistant (a fellow graduate student) who was hired to transcribe the interviews. This contributed to the next level of analysis, where the first stages of emerging themes were discussed between the transcriber and me. I asked participants if they would like a copy of their transcription to review before I started the analysis, and 11 participants agreed. From their feedback I was able to assess the accuracy of their transcriptions and modified the transcripts where necessary. I then reviewed each transcription and started to identify potential topic and issues in the data. These formed the basis of a coding frame, in which I read each transcript and applied the existing frame while looking for new topics that could be added to the coding frame. I read the transcripts a final time to examine how topics were related and to establish linkages between topics in the coding frame. I used a spreadsheet to identify key themes and to keep count of the individual themes as they were mentioned in the participants' responses. The spreadsheet was designed to easily convey the emerging codes and main themes in a quantifiable manner to the purposes of the research team, and could therefore be accessible for use with the larger research project. Data collected from these interviews for this research provided 'snapshots' of women's experiences with risk perception and categorisation.

Findings

Health and social care professionals as adversaries and allies

The majority of women I interviewed did not access maternity care until they were five or six months pregnant, either because they had only become aware they were pregnant several months into their pregnancy or because they were concerned about possible negative of judgement by health and social care professionals.

Six of the women felt that health and social services had been critical or unsupportive. Underpinning these women's accounts was a perception that they were not taken seriously or given respect by services. For example, Jessie indicated that her midwife was not willing to support her request for a home birth. She noted that 'my midwife I'm not appreciating so much right now, 'cause she's doubting my homebirth'. While Jessie stated that she was aware that her midwife was concerned about a number of risk factors including Jessie's lack of parental support and stable housing and history of drug misuse, Jessie felt that her midwife was not listening to her desires to have a 'natural' birth, that her choice for her labour and delivery was not being taken seriously. Shelby noted the ways in which current services disregarded her special circumstances and that she 'just didn't have the supports as far as an addiction and being a young mom'. She also expressed concern that if she lapsed during pregnancy and started using then the services would withdraw all support:

if I had slipped, I don't think that there would've been any help for me as a new mom.

Thus several of the participants in the study noted that health and social care professionals were unwilling to engage with them if they became aware of their risk-taking behaviours such as drug use during pregnancy, or, if they started using again during pregnancy.

For seven of the participants in my study this lack of engagement and respect was reflected in perceived lack of choice throughout their pregnancy and delivery. Rose described her lack of choice she had during her first pregnancy, when she had been using drugs:

> With my first I was nineteen and I was, had no idea what I was doing and I would've done it a lot different. It was very, very medical, very, very by the books and I had a birth plan written out that was a natural birth plan and it was kind of scoffed at by all of the professionals once I got to the hospital. So, but [I]didn't really have a choice.

Most of the mothers felt they were treated as high risk and subject to heightened surveillance during their pregnancy. For example, eight women said that they had been regularly drug tested during their pregnancy, and they were not given a choice about such tests. Some women said they were happy with this increased surveillance as they could show they were not taking drugs while they were pregnant. For example, Becca described the testing regime of the doctor who supervised her pregnancy in the following way:

> Pretty much right away [the doctor] instated um, weekly random drug tests, which I was fine with because that way I knew that if anything came up anybody called in on me, if there's any type of problems I could down on paper with the nurse standing over me watching me urinate that I hadn't been doing drugs.

Elena described how she felt compelled to comply with drug testing so she could keep her child:

> I had to do random drug testing uh, which was pretty much, it was voluntary for me, 'cause I wanted to keep her [daughter].

Most of the women in my study understood and accepted to varying degrees of risk management in order to retain custody of their children after their birth. They accepted random drug testing during pregnancy as a way of managing risk, in this case the risk of losing their child if they did not prove to officials that they were responsible mothers who could control their drug use to protect their foetus.

However, in their interviews the women also commented on the hassle and anxiety created by regular drug tested during pregnancy. For example, Shelby described the ways in which drug testing disrupted her life:

> At first it was, um, I had to call into a number uh, every single day, um, for about three, I think it was three, in three-month increments. Um, and they would tell me yes or no that, that day right when then and there you'd come in at this time. And automatic fail if you don't show up.

This meant that official representatives of the health ministry played a major role in these women's lives and that the threat of losing care of their children loomed large and engendered an atmosphere of distrust and fear towards a government institution that was initially created to monitor the welfare of children and families. Such an environment did little to promote cooperation with official from the Ministry of Child and Family Development in the early years of the lives of these women's children.

Eleven women stated that the Ministry of Child and Family Development played an important part in their lives. They referred to it as 'the Ministry', 'social services' or simply their 'social worker'. Participants expressed how important it was to know that their case file with Ministry of Child and Family Development was closed. Laura expressed frustration that her meticulous actions to avoid Ministry involvement were fruitless, as an anonymous person reported her to the Ministry the day after her child was born. The report claimed she was drinking alcohol during pregnancy, an accusation that she adamantly denied. She successfully retained custody of her child as random drug testing results during her pregnancy and after the birth of her child had all been negative.

Nine participants said that when they became pregnant they were worried that their child might be removed from their care after birth. They noted how this anxiety acted as a barrier to accessing health and social services. Rose recognised that professionals had a child protection duty and an obligation to report any harmful situations such as drug use by a mother that might place a child at risk:

> It was really, really, really stressful cause I didn't feel like I could talk to anybody about it.

Elena described a tense situation between her and a Ministry worker:

> They [the Ministry workers] basically told me that if there was any drugs found in her [daughter's] system, she was drug tested right at birth, at birth um, if, then if there was any drugs in her system aside from the ones that they gave him and went to her um, that she would be taken from me immediately and there was nothing in her system, obviously; she's here with me.

The fear of the perceived risk of child removal was so great for some of the women I interviewed that even if they accessed maternity services, they were unwilling to disclose their entire history of adverse health behaviours to their provider. Melissa explained that she

> Was honest with her [midwife] to a point about my [substance] usage [of crack cocaine], but as far as she knows I stayed clean as soon as I found out 'cause I didn't tell hardly anybody because I was afraid of the Ministry of Children services coming down on me.

Judy also said she was economical with the truth:

> I think there's always the risk hanging over people's head *if they're too honest, they're gonna deal with social workers* (italics added).

Women's awareness of the dangers of intervention in their lives meant that they were reluctant to disclose their health behaviours and communicate their needs during their pregnancy. Some women such as Veronica felt they had a duty to disclose all relevant information. She said that she

> was pretty honest with her [obstetrician] about everything. I mean I thought that's my duty as a pregnant woman to do for my child so that she could give me the best care.

However Veronica's response was exceptional, most women in the study feared that if they fully disclosed their child would be taken from them. For example, Shelby stated that:

> not being perfect in their [social services] eyes meant that I couldn't have my daughter.

Some of the women in the study said they were unwilling to discuss mental health issues with service providers such issues were not addressed during their pregnancy. Elena described this in her interview in the following way:

Had post partum depression for two years so I would've liked some counselling, but I just didn't know how to ask I guess. I just didn't wanna, I didn't wanna bother people with my problems I guess [...] I was scared that because I had had the Ministry involved already for um, the drugs and drinking while I was pregnant that someone would be like 'oh, well she's unstable to take care of her child' or something like that, so I just didn't ask, cause I just was scared.

Elena's fear that service providers would consider her not fit to look after her child if she told her she had mental health issues in addition to her drinking and drug use problems, which the services were aware of, meant that she did not discuss them and did not receive the post-natal mental health care she needed.

Five women who I interviewed had their children removed from their care shortly after they gave birth. Clara told a grim story about her anguish of not being able to breastfeed, and subsequently not bonding with her daughter, after her child was removed from her care. Clara did not have a stable home and lived in a motel, saving her pumped breast milk in her hotel fridge in the hope of regaining custody over her child and being able to breastfeed. Clara described how

I had the health nurse come because I was, bloating up and it was really bad and I, and then my, my milk wasn't coming in for a while so they suggested smelling her clothes, so the clothes that I had her in, in the hospital. So here I am in a motel, smelling a baby's clothes [...] that was a big heartbreak for me. And uh, I think she missed out on it, and the whole time I was pregnant with her, everybody, about how important it is breast milk and blah blah blah, all through the pregnancy and uh, had me really excited about doing it. And I missed out. Missed out on it; something I'll never get back.

Clara's experience demonstrates the impact of decisions by health and social services on these women's lives. Clara was aware as a result of public health campaigns that breastfeeding is the healthiest option for a new baby, but experienced distress as she was unable to fulfil this need. She was homeless, living in temporary accommodation in an area that was prone to, in Clara's words: 'drug dealers and addicts' while she was dealing with depression over the removal of her child.

Risk internalised as stigma

Nine of the women I interviewed said that they felt that stigmatised. These nine women expressed feeling of shame, guilt, and other negative emotions about their drug use. All women were aware that using drugs during their pregnancy could affect their babies' development, and expressed guilt and self-loathing during and after their drug use. In their interviews some suggested that these feeling contributed to a cycle of using drugs to find relief from life stressors, only to feel bad about their use and ultimately add to their stress with pressure for more drug use.

Twelve women said they recognised the stigma associated with drug use during pregnancy. For example, Rose stated that:

I don't think there's really anything that people hate as much as like, a pregnant woman who uses drugs.

Elena suggested that as she was categorised as a 'drug-using mother' her behaviour was always and continually exposed to moral scrutiny:

> I've had situations um, some of the places where I do feel like even though they're great programmes and I always feel happy that I went, I felt judged or like, I've been taken the wrong way.

The women in the study indicated that this feeling of moral scrutiny deterred them from seeking access to programmes that they felt they could benefit from during their pregnancy. They indicted that this sense of stigma led to a form of self-censorship in which they concealed some of their risk-taking behaviours. Elena said this because people assumed that she was taking risks and she was unwilling to trust them:

> Another thing that's really hard with being pregnant and dealing with any kind of thing, things like that is obviously – the stigma. I think people assume if you're, I think just people assume a lot of bad things, unfortunately. So it can be really hard to feel open enough to want to um, tell people that that's what you're going through and access services.

In their interviews the women indicated that stigma was a major risk factor in their lives in which resulted in interactions with health and social care professionals that were shaped by these professionals' negative and moralising judgements. They said that they responded to such anticipated reactions by limiting their use of these services. However they also indicated that they tended to accept these stigmatising stereotypes of women drug users and this resulted in a loss of self-confidence and an acceptance that their behaviour was irresponsible and harmful. For example, in her interview, Becca accepted that her use of methadone was harmful to her baby. She suggested that she had not planned the pregnancy and that she felt guilty that her baby would be born with withdrawal symptoms:

> I never wanted to have a baby while I was on methadone. I, one of the things that was really hard for me was coming to terms with the fact that my baby might be born with withdrawal symptoms just from being on the methadone.

Most of the women noted that struggling with the guilt of engaging in adverse health behaviours during pregnancy was an ongoing battle, and added to an already stressful situation.

Several of the women referred to their child specifically as a 'blessing' and indicated that their pregnancy was an event that had enabled them to regain control over their lives and to reduce or stop their drug use. Laura stated that: 'I didn't expect to be pregnant. It straightened up my life through. It was a blessing'. Susan, who had issues with drug use during a pregnancy that was nearly 10 years before the interview, reflected on the experience and how it had affected her life. In her interview she described how she explained to her child the impact of the birth:

> [I said to my son] 'You know what if you hadn't come into my life like I would be making bad choices and, and I wouldn't be doing this. Like you're, you're the best gift that, that's ever happened to me'.

In their interviews the women emphasised the central role which their children played in their lives and emphasised the ways they were committed to acting in the best interest of their children by reducing risks they accepted were threats in their children's and their own well-being.

The women in our interview presented themselves as responsible mothers who were committed to reducing risks for their unborn and new-born children, but who found the stigmatisation of their drug use to be a barrier to accessing the services they needed to reduce this risk.

Discussion

In the interviews which I have drawn on in this article I have examined 13 women who used drugs during pregnancy talked about the risks associated with their pregnancy including the potential hazards of interacting with health and social care professionals and government institutions. Health and social care professionals acted as both adversaries and allies, facilitating risk management strategies but also representing a source of risk through moralising attitudes towards the women interviewed for this study. The stigma of using drugs while pregnant, and to a lesser extent the drug use itself, manifested as major risk factors for the women who participated in this study. The effect of such stigmatisation was instrumental in the amount of perceived choice and self-efficacy participants had over risk management in their lives. Some participants were cooperative with the different risk management techniques such as random drug testing; as such measures were proof of their compliance to the dominant public health and social norms of striving to have a drug free pregnancy. However, this form of surveillance also both reinforced and reminded women of the stigmatising label bestowed on them due to their drug use while pregnant, and further perpetuated the putative belief of their failed self-efficacy to be 'a normal pregnant woman'. Such risk management approaches left participants feeling they lacked control over their pregnancies, and had little choice to advocate for the changes they desired.

The concept of risk described by the women in this study often materialised as the ever-present fear of having their child removed from their care. This risk was further exacerbated by the absence of social supports where women could express their fears in a safe, non-judgemental environment. Such lack of support, while consistent with the rhetoric of self-responsibility, acted as counterproductive measures to facilitating risk management techniques pregnant women actually identified as a need (such as counselling). The fear of the Ministry and the scarcity of support to deal with such fear manifested as another source of risk in participants' lives in which the women themselves had limited or no control.

Furthermore, the women in this study described the ways in which potential or actual risks as a condition of their drug use during pregnancy manifested as an internalised form of stigma. Participants subsumed the predominant rhetoric of motherhood to varying degrees, which added to the feelings of guilt and blame already projected on them. Such self-stigmatisation added to participants' lack of autonomy over how risk was identified and managed during their pregnancies.

A distinctive feature of this study was the way in which the women interpreted their drug in terms of different types of risk and risk categorisation. Although the women had a grasp of the structural forces that dictated the risk management techniques used on their pregnant bodies, the stigmatisation of their drug use and their position as a relatively marginalised population resulted in an inability to effectively resist the debilitating effect such moralising beliefs. The findings from this study contribute not only to highlighting the ambiguous tension between individual and structural understandings of risk categorisation and management, but also emphasise the detrimental role both external and internal stigmatisation plays in the lives of pregnant women who use drugs.

Conclusion

In this article, I have examined the ways in 13 women who used drugs during their pregnancy discussed the risk and their interactions with services. The women indicated that they experienced stigmatising attitudes from health and social care professionals and government institutions in the form of 'risk management', and that the internalisation of this stigma, resulted in a decrease of self-efficacy and ultimate worse outcomes for participants' well-being. Stigmatisation not only perpetuated health-related risks in the women interviewed for this study; participants realised that stigmatisation is one of the crucial risk factors in their lives while they were pregnant. Such stigmatisation added to and complicated already difficult situations in participants' lives, and resulted in exacerbating rather than decreasing women's risk factors. The participants in the study often internalised this understanding of risk and this manifested itself in delays in accessing maternal health and social care services. The women in the study had different understandings of risk and these were structured by the women's own understanding of the general risk factors during their pregnancy, as well as their experiences of the constructions of risk and risk management by health and social care professionals. While structural life chances can constrain women's feelings of self-efficacy, services that promote clients' ability to make choices can facilitate reduced stigmatisation and facilitate the development of more compassionate and autonomous approaches to risk management.

Acknowledgements

I would like to thank the individuals at the Centre for Addictions Research British Columbia, the University of Victoria, and the women who participated in this research project.

Notes

1. The author of this article was sole interviewer for this research, as the fieldwork and data analysis were part of the academic requirements for obtaining a Master of Arts degree in Sociology. The researchers who were involved with the larger research project were comprised of nurses, academics, medical doctors and community representatives who worked together with the HerWay Home Programme planning team and main funders to develop the programme from the initial conception, design and eventual delivery. Professor Cecilia Benoit supervised this Masters research and was the principal investigator of the larger research project.
2. This research was funded by the Banting and Charles Best Canada Graduate Scholarship, granted by the Canadian Institute for Health Research, and through a fellowship from the Sarah Spencer Foundation.

References

Beck, U., 1992. *Risk society: toward a new modernity*. London: Sage Publishing.
Benoit, C., Shumak, L., and Barlee, D., 2010. *Stigma and health of vulnerable women*. Research Brief 2. [online] The Women's Health Research Network. Available from: www.whrn.ca/documents/Stigma.pdf. [Accessed 15 March 2010].
Boyd, S., 1999. *Mothers and illicit drugs: transcending the myths*. Toronto: University of Toronto Press.
Boyd, S., 2001. Feminist research on others and illegal drugs. *Resources for feminist research*, 28 (3/4), 113–130.
Burton-Jeangros, C., 2011. Surveillance of risks in everyday life: the agency of pregnant women and its limitations. *Social theory and health*, 9 (4), 419–436.
Butler, J., 1990. *Gender trouble: feminism and the subversion of identity*. London: Routledge.
Campbell, N., 2000. *Using women: gender, drug policy, and social justice*. London: Routledge.

Campbell, N. and Ettorre, E., 2011. *Gendering addiction: the politics of drug treatment in a neurochemical world*. Basingstoke: Palgrave Macmillian.

Charmaz, K., 2008. Grounded theory in the 21st century: applications for advancing social justice studies. *In*: N. Denzin and Y. Lincon, eds. *Strategies of qualitative inquiry*. London: Sage Publishing, 203–242.

Charmaz, K. and Mitchell, G., 2001. Grounded theory. *In*: P. Atkinson, A. Coffey and S. Delamont eds. *Handbook of ethnography*. London: Sage Publishing, 128–153.

Collingridge, D. and Gantt, E., 2008. The quality of qualitative research. *American journal of medical quality*, 23, 389–395.

Davis, K. and Yonkers, K., 2012. Making lemonade out of lemons: a case report an literature review of external pressure as an intervention with pregnant and parenting substance-using women. *Journal of clinical psychiatry*, 73 (1), 51–56.

Davoren, J. and Poag, B., 2010. *Her way home program: comprehensive programming for women and children in Victoria* [PowerPoint slides]. [online]. Available from: http://search.phsa.ca/cgi-bin/MsmGo.exe?grab_id=0&page_id=9596&query=herway%20home%20program [Accessed 5 December 2013].

Ettorre, E., 2004. Revisioning women and drug use: gender sensitivity, embodiment and reducing harm. *International journal of drug policy*, 15 (5–6), 327–335.

Friedman, S., Heneghan, A., and Rosenthal, M., 2009. Characteristics of women who do not seek prenatal care and implications for prevention. *Journal of obstetric gynaecologic and neonatal nursing*, 38, 174–181.

Glaser, B. and Strauss, A., 1967. *The discovery of grounded theory: strategies for qualitative research*. Chicago, IL: Aldine.

Goffman, E., 1963. *Stigma: notes on the management of spoiled identity*. London: Penguin Group.

Greaves, L. and Poole, N., 2008. Highs and lows: Canadian perspectives on women and substance use. *Canadian women's health network*, 10 (2), 29–33.

Humphries, D., 1999. *Crack mothers: pregnancy, drugs and the media*. Columbia, MO: Ohio State University Press.

Leslie, M. and DeMarchi, G., 2004. Engaging pregnant women using substances: review of the Breaking the Cycle pregnancy outreach program. *IMPrint: newsletter of the infant mental health promotion project*, 39, 1–5.

Link, B. and Phelan, J., 2001. Conceptualizing stigma. *Annual review of sociology*, 27, 363–385.

Link, B. and Phelan, J., 2006. Stigma and its public health implications. *Lancet*, 367, 528–529.

Lupton, D., 2012. Precious cargo': foetal subjects, risk and reproductive citizenship. *Critical public health*, 22 (3), 239–340.

Macrory, F. and Boyd, S., 2007. Developing primary and secondary services for drug and alcohol dependent mothers. *Seminars in foetal & neonatal medicine*, 12, 119–126.

Marcellus, L., 2004. Feminist ethics must inform practice: interventions with perinatal substance users. *Health care for women international*, 25, 730–742.

Marshall, S., *et al.*, 2005. Sheway's services for substance using pregnant and parenting women: evaluating the outcomes for infants. *Canadian journal of community mental health*, 24 (1), 19–33.

Pinkham, S. and Malinowska-Sempruch, K., 2007. *Women, harm reduction, and HIV*. New York: Open Society Institute.

Poole, N. and Isaac, B., 2001. *Apprehensions: barriers to treatment for substance-using mothers*. Vancouver, WA: British Columbia Centre of Excellence for Women's Health.

Radcliffe, P., 2011. Substance-misusing women : Stigma in the maternity setting. *British journal of midwifery*, 19 (8), 497–606.

Rutman, D., *et al.*, 2000. *Substance use and pregnancy: conceiving women in the policy making process*. Ottawa: Status of Women Canada.

Salmon, A., 2011. Aboriginal mothering, FASD prevention and the contestations of neoliberal citizenship. *Critical public health*, 21 (2), 165–178.

Stubber, J. and Myer, I., 2008. Stigma, prejudice, discrimination and health. *Social science and medicine*, 67, 351–357.

Sword, W., Niccols, A., and Fan, A., 2004. 'New Choices' for women with addictions: perceptions of program participants. *BMC public health*, 4, 10–20.

Tulloch, J. and Lupton, D., 2003. *Risk and everyday life*. London: Sage Publications.

Uziel-Miller, N. and Lyons, J., 2000. Specialized substance abuse treatment for women and their children: an analysis of program design. *Journal of substance abuse treatment*, 19, 355–367.

Woolgar, S. and Pawluch, D., 1985. Ontological gerrymandering: the anatomy of social problems explanations. *Social problems*, 32 (3), 214–227.

Young, I., 1994. Punishment, treatment, empowerment: three approaches to policy for pregnant addicts. *Feminist studies*, 20 (1), 33–57.

'Why take chances?' Advice on alcohol intake to pregnant and non-pregnant women in four Nordic countries

Anna Leppo[a], Dorte Hecksher[b] and Kalle Tryggvesson[c]

[a]Department of Social Research, University of Helsinki, Helsinki, Finland; [b]Department of Forensic Psychiatry, Aarhus University Hospital, Risskov, Denmark; [c]Department of Criminology, University of Stockholm, Stockholm, Sweden

In this article we explore the construction of risk in government guidelines on alcohol intake during and before pregnancy in four Nordic countries given that there is no sound evidence linking a low level of alcohol intake during pregnancy to foetal harm. In the article we draw on two sources of data to examine the rationale behind the advice given to pregnant women: health education materials and other government documents, such as guidelines for professionals. We found that in all the four countries the government guidelines advised pregnant women to completely abstain from alcohol consumption, but there was some variation between the countries in the advice for non-pregnant women. The guidance in the four countries also differed in the extent to which they discussed the lack of evidence behind the abstinence advice and the precautionary approach on which the advice was based. In all the four countries the printed and widely circulated health education materials did not explain that the abstinence advice was not based on actual evidence of harm but on a precautionary approach. The other government documents adopted varying strategies for justifying the abstinence advice including not offering information about the uncertainty of the knowledge base, implying that there was evidence that low alcohol consumption was harmful to the foetus, acknowledging that a safe level of alcohol intake during pregnancy could not be specified and explaining the precautionary approach to risk. In this article we argue that the shift from 'estimation of risk' to the 'precautionary principle' is a part of a wider socio-cultural push towards broader employment of the precautionary principle as a strategy to manage uncertainty, and in the context of pregnancy, it is a part of the symbolic struggle to protect the purity of the foetus and construct the 'perfect mother'.

Introduction

In contemporary western societies, experts, such as health professionals, show a keen interest in matters related to mothers' and pregnant women's health and lifestyle and women are easily condemned for behaviours that may pose a risk to the foetus or child (Kukla, 2010; Lupton, 2011, 2012; Oakley, 1989). For instance, Rothman (2014) notes that the language of risk has completely invaded pregnancy. This socio-cultural climate makes the question of alcohol, pregnancy and regulation of risk a pertinent topic for sociological inquiry. In this article we examine the construction of risk and management of uncertainty in government guidelines and documents on alcohol intake during pregnancy in four Nordic countries.

Alcohol, pregnancy and risk

In the early 1970s medical researchers identified birth abnormalities found in children born to alcoholic women and labelled the phenomenon foetal alcohol syndrome (Golden, 2005). More recently such experts have suggested that low-to-moderate alcohol intake may also cause foetal harm and have coined the term 'foetal alcohol spectrum disorder' to refer a wide range of permanent birth defects which may be caused by alcohol. Foetal alcohol spectrum disorder includes foetal alcohol syndrome and other less severe foetal abnormalities (Golden, 2005; Sokol, Delaney-Black, & Nordstrom, 2003). Gray, Mukherjee, and Rutter (2009) argued that while it is clear that heavy alcohol consumption can result in foetal alcohol syndrome, the effects of drinking at low-to-moderate[1] levels are much less clear. O'Leary and Bower (2011) concluded that while the risk of harm was well documented with heavy and moderate levels of exposure, there was no strong research evidence of adverse effects from low levels of alcohol exposure (see also Hendersson, Gray, & Brocklehurst, 2007).[2] When we were reviewing the literature for this article in 2011 and 2012, we could find no consistent evidence linking a low level of alcohol use during pregnancy to adverse effects.[3] However as we will show in this article it has become increasingly common for the public health authorities to urge women not to consume any alcohol during pregnancy or if they are 'trying to conceive'. In this article we examine how this development can be understood and explained.

Risk and morality

In this article we use a constructionist approach to risk which highlights the socio-cultural aspects of risk and asks how risks are constructed as being real (Zinn, 2009). Technical approaches to risk assume that there are objective measureable and calcul-able risks, while sociological studies of risk highlight the ways in which risks are socially moulded and negotiated: some hazards and harm are not socially relevant even though they have huge consequences for masses of people while others become prominent even though there is little or no evidence that they exist (Zinn, 2009). The constructionist approach to risk focuses on a range of ways in which people, organisa-tions or societies deal with uncertain futures and the very notion of risk is linked to the modern idea that we are responsible for our future and can do something about it (Zinn, 2009).

In order to understand the debates on risk, alcohol and pregnancy, it is important to be aware that concepts of morality underpin and are embedded in risk. According to Douglas (1992, 29), debate on risk 'links some real danger and some disapproved behaviour, coding the danger in terms of a threat to a valued institution'. For Douglas, selection between different potential risks is always a political and moral issue, and in many cases the term 'danger' would in fact be more apt than 'risk' as decisions about which risks are highlighted, are not made solely on the basis of probability calculations and scientific evidence even when such evidence is available. Douglas (1992) argued that 'risk' has become a popular conceptualisation for dangers and uncertainties because it carries the aura of scientific objectivity which to some extent conceals its moral underpinnings. Douglas underlined the nature of risk as moral danger that binds a community together and draws its boundaries and values (Douglas & Wildavsky, 1982). In other words, in order for a given danger to be viewed as a major risk, it needs to be viewed as pollution, as a threat to purity.

Drinking alcohol as a risk and moral failing

The identification of all alcohol consumption as a risk can be traced back to the US Surgeon General recommendation in 1981 that pregnant women should not drink alcohol (Armstrong, 2003, p. 90). In 1988 the US Congress passed legislation which specified that alcohol should only be sold in containers that contained a health warning that pregnant women should not drink alcohol.

These decisions were criticised by researchers. For example Plant (1997, pp. 160–163) asked why US Surgeon General had decided to issue this recommendation when current scientific evidence indicated that only heavy drinking was dangerous during pregnancy, and Kaskutas (1995) criticised the US congress legislation on the same grounds. Commentators have suggested that concerns about women's drinking in the United States reflect anxieties about the impact of alcohol on American society and were linked to the perceived increase in child abuse (Armstrong & Abel, 2002) and anxiety about women's role in society (Armstrong, 2003). Thus the concern about women's drinking can be seen as part of a moral panic (Cohen, 1972).

Several researchers have examined government guidelines on alcohol and pregnancy. O'Leary, Heuzenroeder, Elliot, and Bower (2007) compared government alcohol and pregnancy policies and clinical practice guidelines in seven English-speaking countries and found substantial variation. For example, Australian advice at the time was that 'abstinence may be considered' (O'Leary et al., 2007, p. 466), and if a woman did drink, she should not consume more than seven standard drinks a week and no more than two standard drinks on any one day. UK official advice was similar, but, in both the United States and New Zealand, the government called for complete abstinence. In the other countries (Canada, South Africa, Ireland) the official advice was that pregnant women should abstain, but the message was more complex than a simple abstinence message. There was little evidence that the advice was grounded on evidence, only the UK government had commissioned a systematic review of scientific literature and used this to inform the guidelines for pregnant women (O'Leary et al., 2007, p. 467).

Recently both Australia and the United Kingdom have fallen in-line with other English-speaking countries and issued advice based on full abstinence from drinking during pregnancy (Keane, 2013; Lowe & Lee, 2010). In 2007, the English Department of Health issued new advice that pregnant women and 'those trying to conceive' should not drink. However the advice further stated that if a pregnant woman chooses to drink, she should minimise risks by not drinking more than one to two units of alcohol once or twice a week and should not get drunk (Lowe & Lee, 2010, p. 301). Lowe and Lee (2010, p. 306) noted that a review of evidence commissioned by the Department of Health in 2005 found no strong evidence of harmful effects of low-to-moderate intake (less than 1.5 standard units a day) or 'binge drinking' (five or more drinks on one occasion). The English National Institute for Health and Care Excellence (NICE) an arms-length government agency that commissions evidence-based reviews and issues guidance based on them initially used this review to justify encouraging abstinence but also indicating a maximum reasonable level of drinking. However, without any new evidence NICE changed the message to total abstinence in order to send 'a clear message' (Lowe & Lee, 2010, p. 306). Gavaghan (2009, p. 301) criticised the adoption of a total abstinence message in the United Kingdom, labelling it old-fashioned and paternalistic while Lowe and Lee (2010) characterised it as a mechanism for dealing with the uncertainty associated with evidence.

There is also evidence that public agencies in other developed countries have adopted the same approach. Leppo and Hecksher (2011) reported that the Finnish and Danish governments launched total abstinence messages in 2006 and 2007, respectively, and also advised 'women planning pregnancy' not to drink alcohol. Both the countries launched the abstinence message despite the fact that there was no evidence of harm from low alcohol intake. Leppo and Hecksher (2011) argued that a process of international diffusion of total abstinence policy was taking place. However Drabble et al. (2011) have indicated that the diffusion of the abstinence message may be restricted to developed countries, and three non-developed countries in their comparative study did not have formal foetal alcohol spectrum disorder prevention strategies or intervention plans.

Most of the studies of the development of strategies to identify and manage the risks associated with drinking in pregnancy have been in English-speaking countries and have not explored the ways in which health education messages such as abstinence relate to evidence. In this article we will examine how government guidelines and advice on alcohol intake during pregnancy have developed in the four mainland Nordic countries – Denmark, Finland, Sweden and Norway. In this article we use two data sets to analyse how risk communication to the general public differs from communicating risks between experts and professionals. We examine how government health agencies chose to deal with lack of evidence of harm when they communicate the dangers of low alcohol intake during (and before) pregnancy to the general public and to professionals. The Nordic countries, which have a long tradition of developing health and social policies in close proximity, are an interesting case for a comparison, and we examine whether they have followed the same trajectory and copied policy from each other and whether they have adopted equally paternalistic or non-paternalistic approaches and guidelines and relied on a similar precautionary logic.

Methods

Content analysis of key documents

Our primary interest in this article lies in the construction of risk and management of uncertainty in expert discourses on alcohol intake during pregnancy. We are interested in how health experts have chosen to communicate risks to lay people and to other experts and professionals. In order to examine these questions we draw on data from a study in which we collected and analysed government guidelines in four Nordic countries on pregnant women's alcohol intake and collected and analysed related government documents that provided evidence and the rationale for or informed the guidelines. We collected most of these documents in 2011 and some additional documents in 2012. All key documents from each country were included in order to ensure a comprehensive analysis. Documents are a somewhat underused resource in health research, and the use of unsolicited documents is useful for instance in that they are usually relatively easily accessible, they help to access data that are difficult to obtain in other ways, and the researcher does not directly influence the formation of data (Alaszewski, 2013).

Denmark, Finland, Norway and Sweden are Nordic welfare states with a free-of-charge, public maternity care service system which reaches virtually all pregnant women at an early stage of pregnancy and throughout the pregnancy. Printed booklets with information about different aspects of pregnancy are produced by government officials and provided to pregnant women at maternity clinics by general practitioners, nurses or midwives. These printed health education booklets thus reach virtually all pregnant women.

To identify current government advice we initially collected the most recent health education booklets that contained advice and recommendations on pregnant women's alcohol intake. All the booklets we collected and examined were available both in printed format and online and had been translated into other languages. We used the original versions and English translations. In all the countries except Finland, the government had public health websites which had information and advice on pregnancy and drinking, and we downloaded and included relevant material in our data set.

These public health booklets and websites are designed to provide the general public including pregnant women with information and advice. There was also more specialist and technical documentation designed to inform policy decisions or to provide professionals caring for and advising pregnant women with up-to-date evidence. These documents included research reviews produced and commissioned by government officials, policy documents and guidelines for professionals. We identified the most important and recent documents from each country and included them in our data set.

Data analysis

Two of the researches (Anna Leppo and Dorte Hecksher) started the analysis by reading all the Finnish and Danish documents several times and then discussing their initial impressions. Based on our review of previous literature and our reading of the data, we agreed to focus on three major themes in the documents: whether it promoted abstinence or not, how the advice/guidance was justified (in particular if scientific evidence of risk was cited) and whether the precautionary approach was explicitly mentioned or explained. Once we had agreed on these themes, all the three authors read the documents identifying and coding the relevant material on drinking and pregnancy, and these data form the basis of our findings in this article.

These data cannot be used to explain why a given health education message was adopted in a specific country nor how and why the risks were communicated in this particular format. Such analyses could only be based on data derived from in-depth case studies of this area of public health policy in each country. In this article we focus on the 'outcome' of this complex social, political and scientific process, the part that is visible in the official guidelines and documents.

Findings

We start this Findings section with a country-by-country analysis of relevant documents. We then examine whether there are differences and why this is the case.

Denmark

In Denmark the National Board of Health (Sundhedsstyrelsen) formulates the policy and guidelines on alcohol and pregnancy and is, in collaboration with the Danish Committee for Health Education, responsible for delivering guidelines to health professionals and producing health education material.

From 1998 until 2007 Board advised pregnant women not to drink, but if they drank they were not to drink more than one standard drink on any one day and avoid drinking every day (Leppo & Hecksher, 2011). This advice was based on a systematic review of evidence conducted by an expert group appointed by the Board.

In 2007 the Board of Health replaced its previous, more liberal pregnancy guideline with an abstinence message, and the 2010 edition of its advice to women booklet includes an unequivocal 'no alcohol' message for pregnant mothers and women planning to get pregnant:

> You can prepare for a healthy pregnancy even before you become pregnant..... And stay clear of alcohol and smoking (...) No alcohol. Alcohol can harm your baby from the start of pregnancy and onwards. As it is often difficult to know the exact time of conception, you should not drink alcohol if you are planning on having a baby. (*Healthy habits*, 2010, p. 3)

This message was repeated several times in the booklet in a prescriptive way without any reference to the lack of evidence about the effects of low intakes. For example pregnant women were told to: 'Avoid alcohol and tobacco (...) while you are pregnant (...) alcohol is harmful to the development of the child through the whole pregnancy' (*Healthy habits*, 2010, p. 12). The booklet provided a rationale for its abstinence recommendation citing uncertainty (no exact limit is known) about the effects of alcohol on the foetus as the reason for adopting a precautionary approach:

> If a pregnant woman drinks alcohol, her unborn baby will have the same concentration of alcohol in his or her blood as the mother. The alcohol is absorbed by the woman's blood and passes through the placenta to the baby. Alcohol is harmful to the baby's development throughout pregnancy. *No exact limit is known for how little a pregnant woman can drink without harming her unborn baby.* The recommendation is therefore for pregnant women not to drink any alcohol at all. The harmful effects of alcohol are life-long and depend on how much the woman drinks. The most serious effects are brain damage and heart defects. (*Healthy habits*, 2010, p. 12, our emphasis)

The assumption underlying the health education message is that responsible women who knew they were pregnant would not drink alcohol. For example in their advice to professionals the government noted that maternity care professionals might encounter women who have consumed alcohol before they knew they were pregnant and that in such cases the professionals should conduct 'a balanced risk-evaluation', presumably to assess if there was likely to be foetal damage though this guidance noted that in most cases the likelihood of such harm was small (Sundhedsstyrelsen, 2009, p. 93). Again this assumption of responsible mothering plus the minimisation of risk is evident in the booklet for pregnant women:

> ... if you find that you are pregnant without having planned it, and you have been drinking alcohol, it is rarely cause for concern. You may like to talk to your doctor/midwife about this when going for your first consultation. (*Healthy habits*, 2010, p. 3)

The booklet for pregnant mothers did note there was a lack of evidence of risk about the effects of low-to-moderate intake of alcohol on the foetus, but did not explain how and why it was advocating a precautionary approach to this uncertainty. In contrast the information intended for professionals did explicitly discuss what the precautionary principle means and why it was adopted (Sundhedsstyrelsen, 2009, pp. 92–93). In a document from 2009 that is available on the Board of Health website on alcohol and pregnancy, it was stated the abstinence message was based on the precautionary principle since the scientific literature on the subject was ambiguous (Den bedste start, 2009).

In Denmark the Board of Health justified its adoption of the principle of total abstinence in 2007 and its shift from the rationale of interpreting risks from 'estimation of risk' to 'principle of caution' on the basis of scientific uncertainty. The new abstinence message was designed to make both the Board and the mothers safer and more responsible (Leppo & Hecksher, 2011; Strandberg-Larsen & Grønbæk, 2006).

Finland

In Finland the National Institute for Health and Welfare (Terveyden ja hyvinvoinnin laitos, THL) regularly republishes a booklet to pregnant women with information and advice on pregnancy, health and parenting which contains short section on alcohol. Since 2006 the booklet has advised pregnant women to abstain from drinking alcohol. The 2010 edition included the following statement:

> Alcohol causes foetal damage. When a pregnant woman drinks alcohol, so does her foetus, because alcohol passes through the placenta and travels via the umbilical cord into the foetus. The blood alcohol level can be higher in the foetus than in the mother. (…) Binge drinking (consuming large quantities of alcoholic beverages) is particularly dangerous for the foetus. The body parts and organs develop during the first trimester (…) and a dangerous drinking pattern during the first trimester can result in foetal malformations, for example a congenital heart defect. Excessive alcohol use should be avoided whenever there is a possibility of pregnancy. Pregnant women should avoid alcohol completely. Alcohol slows down foetal growth throughout the pregnancy and may result in low birth weight. The foetal central nervous system (CNS) is very vulnerable, and at worst the baby may suffer from mental retardation. Alcohol-related foetal defects may cause problems associated with attention span, learning, and linguistic development. *There is no safe amount of alcohol that a woman can drink while pregnant.* Excessive alcohol consumption during pregnancy increases the risk of miscarriage. Other risks include (…). (We're having a baby, 2009, pp. 17–18, our emphasis)

This booklet claimed there was a direct causal link between alcohol consumption and harm to the foetus so that even the smallest amount of alcohol would damage the foetus. Giving a long list of adverse outcomes served to create an impression that all drinking whether low-to-moderate or heavy was dangerous. The advice has given the aura of scientific certainty using technical terms such as the foetal central nervous system (CNS) and alcohol-related foetal defects. There is no acknowledgement of the uncertainty and lack of scientific evidence about the effects on low levels of drinking.

In the advice to and guidelines for health professionals, there is a differentiation between the risks of low and high consumption and an acknowledgement of the uncertainty around and the lack of scientific evidence about the effects of low alcohol consumption. However this uncertainty is used to justify the precautionary abstention approach, the 'better safe than sorry' approach:

> A safe drinking level of alcohol use with regards to malfunction of the central nervous system is not known, and the safest choice during pregnancy is abstinence 'Current care guidelines: Treatment of alcohol abuse 2005'. It is safest to start abstinence already when planning pregnancy. (Sosiaali – ja terveysministeriö, 2007, p. 67)

These guidelines for professionals justified the abstinence policy in terms of uncertainty; the lack of knowledge about a safe drinking level. Unlike Denmark, the Finnish guidelines did not explain or justify its precautionary approach. These guidelines also referred to the overarching national Current Care Guidelines based on evidence-based care and treatment. In the Current Care document there was as short statement that 'Pregnant women are advised to abstain and getting drunk is particularly risky' but no discussion about the precautionary principle or explanation that the abstinence advice was not based on evidence of harm but on an expert judgement and a decision to apply the precautionary principle (Käypä hoito, 2012).

Norway[4]

In Norway the Directorate of Health, Department of Health (the Helsedirektoratet) had several media campaigns aimed at reducing alcohol consumption during pregnancy and its latest guidance; a short health education booklet was published in 2009 (The Best Start Possible, 2009). The booklet had two themes; information and advice about alcohol during pregnancy and how to avoid drinking while pregnant. The booklet stated that any alcohol consumption during pregnancy would harm the baby:

> Research has shown that alcohol can affect the development of the baby's brain and other organs even when drunk in very small quantities. (The best start..., column 1)

The booklet used this 'causal' link between drinking and foetal harm to prescribe total abstention. Mothers should not 'take any chances' with the well-being of their unborn baby. While the key statement in the following extract starts as a recommendation the key verb is an instruction linking to the moral imperative of giving 'your child the best possible start in life':

> It is impossible to quote any definite lower threshold figure for the amount of alcohol a baby can tolerate. It is however a fact that vulnerability varies from foetus to foetus. This is why *we recommend that you do not take any chances – instead you should abstain from drinking alcohol during pregnancy. By doing so you will give your child the best possible start in life.* (The best start..., columns 1–2, our emphasis)

The booklet focuses on alcohol and gives an unequivocal abstinence message which is justified by stating that research shows that alcohol can have an adverse effect on the foetus 'even when drunk in very small quantities'. The booklet does not mention or discuss the uncertainties about the effect of low-to-moderate consumption. The booklet also categorises women planning pregnancy in the risk category and advices them that 'the wisest thing is to change your drinking habits when you are planning to have a child' (The best start..., columns 2–3).

In Norway the abstinence message was preceded by advice issued by the National Institute for Alcohol and Drug Research and the state-owned Wine and Spirit Monopoly which stated that drinking low quantities of alcohol was not likely to have harmful effects on the foetus. In 2004 the Department of Health appointed an expert group to review the scientific evidence on the effect of prenatal alcohol intake on the foetus (Sosial – og helsedirektoratet, 2005a). In its 2005 report the expert group concluded that there was no evidence identifying a safe lower limit for alcohol intake during pregnancy, and therefore, the government should recommend total abstinence for both pregnant women and women planning to get pregnant (Sosial – og helsedirektoratet, 2005a, p. 8).

In 2005 the Department of Health published national guidelines for antenatal care. Although this was a fairly technical document, the foreword indicated that it was hoped that the document would be read by pregnant women as well as professionals. The guidelines included a recommendation that women should not drink during pregnancy, and it would harm the unborn foetus. All the recommendations in the guidelines are linked to an assessment of the evidence which is from 'A' to 'D'. 'A' refers to the strongest possible scientific evidence derived from the gold standard sources of randomised clinical trials while 'D' is the weakest based on expert opinion or clinical practice. In its national guidelines the Department of Health ranks the evidence underpinning the recommendation that women should abstain from drinking while pregnant as the weakest 'D':

> We recommend women not to drink alcohol during pregnancy. [D]. Alcohol has an adverse effect on the foetus. It is advantageous to stop alcohol intake during all stages of pregnancy. [C]. (Sosial – og helsedirektoratet, 2005b, p. 33)

The document did explicitly discuss the evidence underpinning its recommendations. It noted that there were also studies that did not show any adverse effects with low consumption of alcohol (one to two standard drinks per week) (Sosial – og helsedirektoratet, 2005b, p. 79). Given this lack of knowledge, the document justified its recommendations in precautionary, 'better safe than sorry' terms under the heading 'Precautionary principle':

> it is unclear if there is a safe lower limit for prenatal alcohol intake but this does not mean that alcohol intake is not a risk to the foetus and in line with common toxicological and precautionary rationales we advise women to abstain from alcohol during pregnancy. (Sosial – og helsedirektoratet, 2005b, p. 80, our translation)

This reliance on uncertainty as the justification for abstention from low levels of consumptions contrasts with the rationale for advising women to abstain from heavy drinking. In this case of heavy drinking, the document noted there was clear evidence from epidemiological studies that such drinking can cause foetal damage (Sosial – og helsedirektoratet, 2005b, p. 80).

In Norway the rationale for total abstention from drinking during pregnancy recommendation is grounded in the precautionary principle. In developing their guidelines for maternity care professionals, the Norwegian authorities made the decision to conduct their own review of evidence but used the review and grading of evidence conducted in the United Kingdom by NICE in 2003 (Sosial – og helsedirektoratet, 2005b). As we have already noted, NICE did not find any strong evidence of low-to-moderate intake (less than 1.5 standard units a day) was harmful and on the basis of this evidence recommended that health agencies in the United Kingdom should encourage abstinence but also indicate a maximum reasonable level of drinking for pregnant women. The Norwegian authorities reached a different conclusion based on the same evidence.

Sweden

In Sweden two government agencies issue guidelines to pregnant women about alcohol intake. The National Institute of Public Health (the Folkhälsoinstitutet) and the National Food Agency (the Livsmedelsverket) both publish health education material, which is distributed to all pregnant women at prenatal clinics and is also available online.

The National institute for Public Health's booklet focused on alcohol and pregnancy. The booklet's idea and visuals were very similar to the Norwegian booklet in that both made extensive use of ultrasound images of the foetus. It focused on two themes: information and advice about alcohol and how to avoid drinking and provision of information on foetal development. The section dealing with alcohol was prescriptive; it advocated abstention noting the harm that low levels of consumption can cause and advocating a 'better safe than sorry' approach to low levels of consumption:

It is best to abstain from alcohol completely whilst you are pregnant or planning to become pregnant. After a couple of glasses of wine you can have a blood alcohol concentration of 0.5 parts per thousand. The baby is exposed to exactly the same alcohol concentration. The difference is that the baby's cells are much more sensitive. The effects of adding alcohol to cells, how they become disordered or destroyed, can be seen in the laboratory. If you drink alcohol at critical times while the baby is developing important cells then there is a risk that these cells will be damaged (...) The risk of alcohol damage is greatest when you drink large amounts over a long period. *As we don't know what the limits are for the levels of alcohol that can harm the baby, it is safest not to drink alcohol at all during pregnancy.* Studies show that even small amounts of alcohol can result in problems such as hyperactivity, difficulties in concentrating and impaired learning abilities as the child becomes older. (*A good start*, 2009, pp. 2–3, our emphasis)

The target for the abstention advice was both pregnant women and women planning to become pregnant. While the document provides some justification for advice to pregnant women, there is no rationale given for why women planning pregnancy should abstain.

The National Food Agency's booklet for pregnant women was broader in scope and dealt with diet and pregnancy. It did not have any advice about alcohol for women who are planning to get pregnant but did advice pregnant women to abstain. There was a brief justification of this advice:

Alcohol can be transferred to your child via the placenta. The foetus is more sensitive to alcohol than you are, so refrain from alcohol as soon as you believe that you are pregnant. (Advice about food for you who are pregnant, 2008, p. 6)

Both agencies published background material on pregnancy and alcohol including guidelines to professionals. National institute for Public Health's guide for midwives on alcohol and pregnancy contained information about risks of alcohol and provided advice on how to talk with pregnant women about alcohol (Folkhälsöinstitutet, 2009). It recommended that midwives should use Alcohol Use Disorders Identification Test (AUDIT) to assess pregnant women's alcohol consumption. The document stated that the risk of birth defects increased when a woman's consumption exceeded one standard drink per day or seven drinks per week during the first trimester and that intoxication was particularly risky. The document stated that there was no safe level of alcohol intake during pregnancy and advocated abstinence. The guidelines referred to a review of scientific evidence on harm associated with moderate alcohol consumption during pregnancy (Andréasson & Allebeck, 2005), implicitly suggesting that the abstinence advice was based on evidence.

The National Food Agency's guide for midwives was more detailed than their booklet for the women (Livsmedelsverket, 2009). The guidelines concentrated on the most severe harmful effects, namely foetal alcohol syndrome, but failed to mention that this syndrome was caused by a high level of alcohol consumption. However the document did note that there was some evidence that occasional moderate consumption of alcohol early in the pregnancy did not result in harm to the unborn foetus. The document also noted that as it was not known whether low-to-moderate alcohol intake can cause adverse effects to the foetus. The document indicated that midwives should advice pregnant women to abstain from alcohol. Thus the National Food Agency's guidelines were based on the precautionary principle, but its documents did not mention, explain or justify it.

There were contradictions in both the National institute for Public Health's and the National Food Agency's guidelines to professionals. Both indicated that midwives should advise pregnant women to abstain but if a pregnant woman was anxious about having drunk some alcohol, they should seek to reassure them by telling them that drinking a little had probably not harmed their foetus. The 'scientific reviews' about maternal drinking used by both agencies (Göransson & Magnusson, 2005; Livsmedelsverket, 2008) were unsystematic and based on a very limited number of studies, including some with major methodological problems and the reviews chose to focus on the limited number of studies that found adverse effects at the level of 10 grams of alcohol per day or less rather than the larger number that found no adverse effects at such levels. The National Food Agency's 'review of evidence' even mixed references to religious texts (the Bible) about alcohol harms during pregnancy with the modern scientific evidence, highlighting the moral elements embedded in its judgements.

Similarities and differences in the four countries in managing uncertainty

All the health education materials addressed drinking by both pregnant women and those planning to be pregnant. In the case of pregnant women the documents in each country advocated strict abstinence and none of them gave any advice on how pregnant women who did drink could reduce their consumption. This contrasts to the approach in the United Kingdom where women were advised to abstain, but there was also advice for those women 'who choose to drink' on how much alcohol per occasion or week posed 'only a minimal risk' (Lowe & Lee, 2010). The advice for women who planned to become pregnant differed in the four Nordic countries. Danish and Swedish health education material urged women who are 'planning to get pregnant' to abstain, Norwegian guidelines told this group to 'change their drinking habits', with the implication being that they should abstain, while in Finland these women were simply advised 'not to get drunk'.

There were differences between the four countries in how the abstinence message was communicated. In Finland the uncertainty regarding the evidence base of the abstinence message was not communicated to the public. Sweden and Norway provided an ambivalent message, acknowledging that a safe level of alcohol intake was not known but simultaneously claiming that there was evidence of that alcohol was harmful even in 'very small' or 'small' amounts. The Danish material stated that alcohol was harmful to the unborn foetus and that a safe level of alcohol consumption was not known suggesting that a safe level might exist. In none of the four countries did the government health education booklets, which were targeted at and distributed to virtually all pregnant women, explicitly state that there was no unequivocal scientific evidence that low levels of alcohol intake caused harm. All the booklets were based on the assumption that lay reader would not be able to understand complex issues or manage uncertainty; therefore, all the messages were simplified, and the uncertainty removed, but in doing so the booklets provided a misleading message about the risks of low levels of alcohol consumption just before and during pregnancy.

There were differences in the extent to which public health agencies in the different Nordic countries discussed the rationale for their recommendations. In Denmark the online government documents targeted at pregnant women discussed the rationale behind the abstinence advice in detail. The material on the Board of Health website explained what the precautionary principle means and why it had been adopted in Denmark. It acknowledged that there was an alternative for the precautionary principle; the Board could use existing evidence to estimate whether there was evidence that foetuses were harmed by their mothers' low-to-moderate intake and if such evidence did not exist to warn mother about the proven dangers of heavy drinking but not the unproven dangers of low to moderate drinking. In Denmark there has been an expert debate about the precautionary principle in the public fora so that journalists could make references to these debates when reporting on alcohol advice to pregnant women (see for example Jyllands Posten, 2012). In Norway the precautionary principle is only discussed in documents targeted at professionals. However even in these documents there is no debate: precaution is presented as the only option, and it is implied that there is no alternative. In Finland there is no reference to the precautionary principle in material targeted at the public and mothers or professionals. The documents for professionals simply stated that a lower safe drinking level cannot be set and those seeking a justification for the prescription on low to moderate drinking are referred to the Finnish database of evidence based medicine. The implication is that this data base contains evidence justifying the advice on low-to-moderate drinking, but it does not. Finally, in Sweden there is no real discussion of the precautionary principle or of the evidence base. National Institute of Public Health in its advice referenced a review of evidence implying it provided an evidence base for its abstinence advice; however, this source was unsystematic and unreliable. The Swedish Food Safety Agency acknowledged in their guidelines to professionals that it was not known if low-to-moderate alcohol intake can cause adverse effects to the foetus. Their abstinence advice appeared to be based on the precautionary principle, but they did not use, explain or justify the term.

Table 1 sums up the results from the four countries.

Table 1.   Government guidelines on alcohol and pregnancy.

Country	Finland	Sweden	Norway	Denmark
Government agent who issues health education material targeted at pregnant women	National Institute for Health and Welfare (2009)	National Food Agency (2008), National Institute of Public Health (2009)	Directorate of Health (DH) (2009)	National Board of Health (DNBH) (2007)
Guidelines to women planning pregnancy	Advice not to get drunk	National Food Agency: no advice on alcohol to women planning pregnancy National Institute of Public Health: advice to abstain	Advice to change drinking habits	Advice to abstain
Guidelines to pregnant women	Advice to abstain	Advice to abstain	Advice to abstain	Advice to abstain
Rationale behind the advice to pregnant women in the government documents aimed primarily at experts and professionals	Precautionary principle not explicitly mentioned; reference to a review of evidence	Precautionary principle not explicitly mentioned; references to reviews of evidence	Precautionary principle is explicitly mentioned	Precautionary principle is explicitly explained and its justification is discussed

Discussion

Managing uncertainty: from estimation of risk to precaution

Our findings and the evidence from other studies indicate that most developed countries have decided to recommend that women do not drink alcohol when they are pregnant or planning to become pregnant even though there is no systematic evidence indicating that low-to-moderate alcohol intake harms the unborn foetus. Furthermore most of these countries claim that their health policies are based on evidence (Keane, 2013; Leppo & Hecksher, 2011; Lowe & Lee, 2010). The rationale for this ban whether or not it is explicitly stated is precaution, a response to uncertainty in which an outcome is considered so catastrophic that action is taken to mitigate it *irrespective of probability* of it occurring. It therefore differs from conventional risk management that is grounded in evidence about both probability and outcomes. As Alaszewski and Burgess have noted, risk management uses evidence from the past to make decisions in the present to create a better future, whereas the precautionary principle is based on anxieties about the future which shape decisions in the present and are not based on evidence from the past (Alaszewski & Burgess, 2007). These anxieties about 'catastrophic' outcomes are evident in and shape other aspects of the management of pregnancy and childbirth; for example Scamell and Alaszewski (2012) show how midwives focus on the potential harm during birthing and normality is always a post hoc judgement, and Scamell and Stewart (2014) describe how midwives seek to protect themselves from uncertainty and blame by using a rigid timetable to monitor, control and record the birthing process.

The precautionary principle is a particular mode of action in a context of scientific uncertainty: it allows for relaxation of the requirement for causal evidence and justifies risk-preventive actions in the absence of scientific proof (Osimani, 2013). It originated in environmental law to facilitate environmental protection with new types of genetically modified organisms. It reversed the burden of proof in that environmental protection agencies did not need to demonstrate the harm in order to justify prevention but those promoting the new type of organism had to prove that their activities do not cause any serious harm (Osimani, 2013). However the expansion of the precautionary approach to other areas, ones that do not have the same potential for massive environmental catastrophes, has been criticised. Ewald (2002), for instance, has argued that contemporary culture has become increasingly 'riskphobic', and the precautionary principle has become its new regulatory principle.

Room (2005) has noted that very few researchers have tried to establish a safe level of alcohol intake in pregnancy or even examined the effects of occasional drinking (Room, 2005). It is actually very difficult to carry out research on low dose issues (Kesmodel, 2006) and as Gavaghan (2009, p. 300) has noted a positive correlation such as that high doses of alcohol cause foetal damage is relatively easy to demonstrate but the reverse that low doses do not cause harm, negative correlation, is 'notoriously difficult (technically impossible)' to prove.

Lowe and Lee (2010) argued that the adoption of a total abstinence message in the United Kingdom had effectively made uncertainty certain by circumventing uncertainty associated with evidence and simply asserting that it was certain that any alcohol consumption would create harm. A similar circumvention has taken place in all the four countries examined in this article and very recently also in Australia (Keane, 2013). According to Järvinen (2012), studies in other risk communication areas point to parallel processes of transforming the complexity of uncertainty into the simplicity of the precautionary ban.

Gavaghan (2009) has argued that the development of the precautionary approach to pregnancy and alcohol intake is based on old-fashioned paternalism, where experts have decided they know best and have chosen to withhold information that would enable pregnant and prospectively pregnant women to make an informed choice. He suggested that a commitment to honesty and accuracy would involve openly telling pregnant women what the current state of knowledge is and also communicating the uncertainty about the effects of low-to-moderate drinking: it may or may not be harmful. In his view, 'it is not reasonable to replace more accurate information with less accurate merely because it is simpler to communicate' (Gavaghan, 2009, p. 303).

Finally, Gavaghan (2009) fears that issuing advice that may be seen as exaggerating risks may backfire in that the health authorities' advice on other, perhaps more genuine risks, will carry less authority. Of the four Nordic countries studied here, only the Danish health authorities had made an effort to inform pregnant women about the logic behind the abstinence advice.

Protecting the foetus and the all-encompassing demands of motherhood

Adopting the precautionary approach may seem over cautious when engaging in activities that have not been scientifically proven to be totally safe is a normal feature of everyday life (Tryggvesson, 2005). If we practised the precautionary principle in everything we do, we could do very little – and that is what is now asked of pregnant women. The question 'why take chances', posed to pregnant women in the health education material analysed above, suggests paradoxically that a totally risk-free life is a viable option and sends a strong signal that pregnant women and women planning pregnancy should pursue it. There is, however, some evidence that women and clinicians do not accept this risk-averse understanding of prenatal alcohol intake and, in fact, think that an occasional drink does no harm (Hammer & Inglin, 2014).

As Alaszewski (2013, p. 384) notes, babies and young children are seen as particularly susceptible to risk, with parents expected to engage in various strategies of risk-aversion. As numerous studies in the area of constructing risks and social problems have noted, the 'think of the children' argument typically carries significant rhetorical and political weight and is an effective way to mobilise support. For instance, Furedi coined the term 'paranoid parenting' (Furedi, 2002) to refer to the increased concern about safety around children, and Bell (2014) pointed out in connection to the rise of 'third-hand smoke' as a public health issue, that appealing to the safety of children served to give weight to the issue and deflect questions about the degree of harm associated with it. Children are typically viewed as particularly innocent, vulnerable and worthy of keeping safe. Foetuses are even more helpless and thus 'purer' victims, which undoubtedly gives symbolic weight to concerns about their safety.

New medical technologies have in the past decades made the foetus increasingly visible, changing its cultural status and making it into a subject in its own right (Daniels, 1993; Rothman, 1986). For instance, Törrönen and Tryggvesson (2014) have noted how the use of ultrasound images of the foetus in Swedish health education material on alcohol and pregnancy serves to highlight foetal vulnerability. Moreover, underlining the fragility of the foetus and the growing urge to protect foetuses from all potential threats have been identified as current societal trends in the western countries (Bell, McNaughton, & Salmon, 2009; Leppo, 2012; Lupton, 2012).

While the cultural image of the innocent foetus appeals to moral sentiments, two other morally charged cultural images are also intertwined in the case of prenatal alcohol use and its potential harm: that of the perfect mother, who unfailingly keeps her child safe, and the failed mother, who may not follow a precautionary approach to all potential threats, which is, interestingly, framed as 'taking chances'. For instance, Kukla (2010) suggests that the case of drinking in pregnancy is indicative of a larger cultural pattern of holding pregnant women to higher standards of risk management than other people and thinking that pregnant women have a heightened responsibility for risk avoidance. On a symbolic level, the zero-tolerance policy protects not only the purity of the foetus but also of the ideal of the good, if not perfect, mother.

Interestingly, in Australia not only pregnant women and women planning pregnancy but also breast-feeding women have been recently advised to abstain from alcohol, which, according to Keane (2013), manifests a strengthening of the ideology of 'total mother-hood'. The international diffusion of an abstinence message to pregnant women, women planning pregnancy and, most recently, breast-feeding women needs to be understood as a part of a broader cultural shift in which women of a fertile age are expected to devote accumulative action towards maximising foetal and infant health. Women are also expected to start perfecting motherhood earlier than before, even before they become pregnant, and pursue this endeavour for extended periods of time. Interestingly, in this climate, engaging in an activity that has not been scientifically proven to be entirely risk-free can be framed negatively as taking a chance.

Conclusion

In this article we have provided a nuanced analysis of government advice on alcohol intake to pregnant women and women who 'plan to get pregnant' in four mainland Nordic countries: Denmark, Finland, Sweden and Norway. We have shown that the policy regard-ing women 'planning to get pregnant' varies in these countries from advice to abstain to a recommendation not to 'get drunk'. While there is no evidence about the harmfulness of low-level prenatal alcohol intake, pregnant women were advised to abstain in each country. Interestingly, there were different strategies for justifying the abstinence advice: not offering any information regarding the uncertainty of the knowledge base, implying that there is evidence of the harmfulness of low alcohol intake and acknowledging that a safe level of alcohol intake during pregnancy is not known. In none of these countries did the printed and widely circulated health education materials explicitly explain that there was no scientific evidence of any harmful effects of low-level alcohol intake and that the abstinence advice was based on a precautionary approach. In Denmark, however, this logic was communi-cated to the public on a website and to the professionals in other government documents.

Managing uncertainty was not a straightforward task, and this was reflected in the documents we studied which used various strategies to circumvent it especially when communicating risks to lay people. We have argued that the shift from 'estimation of risk' to the 'precautionary principle' in approaching the potential harm of alcohol intake during pregnancy needs to be understood not as an isolated event but as a part of a wider socio-cultural push towards broader employment of the precautionary principle as a strategy to manage uncertainty, especially when children are involved. Moreover, the diffusion of the total abstinence advice should be understood as a symbolic struggle to protect the purity of the foetus and to construct the ideal of the perfect mother.

Acknowledgements

The authors want to thank Karl-Harald Søvig in Norway for his kind and generous assistance in providing data for this article, Nordens Välfärdscenter in Finland for financial assistance for the travel required by the collaboration and the anonymous reviewers of this journal and the editor, Andy Alaszewski, for constructive comments and criticisms.

Notes

1. Low-to-moderate alcohol consumption was defined as maximum 84 grams of alcohol per week, which in the United Kingdom is up to 10.4 'standard units' per week and in the United States up to 7 'standard drinks' per week. The UK standard unit contains 8 grams of alcohol and in the United States 12 grams (Gray et al., 2009).
2. In this study moderate consumption was defined as 30–40 grams of alcohol per occasion and 70 grams per week. In the United Kingdom this would equal 4–5 'standard units' per occasion and almost 9 'standard units' per week.
3. New findings on the effects of low-to-moderate alcohol intake during pregnancy are published all the time. For the purposes of this study it is, however, sufficient to sketch out what was known about the effects of low-to-moderate consumption at the time when the government documents that form the basis of our analysis were published.
4. Karl-Harald Søvig provided the data from Norway.

References

Advice about food for you who are pregnant. (2008). Uppsala: Swedish National Food Administration.
A good start. (2009). Stockholm: The Swedish National Institute of Public Health.
Alaszewski, A. (2013). Vulnerability and risk across the life course. *Health, Risk & Society*, *15*(5), 381–389.
Alaszewski, A., & Burgess, A. (2007). Risk, time and reason. *Health, Risk & Society*, *9*(4), 349–358. doi:10.1080/13698570701612295
Andréasson, S., & Allebeck, P. (Eds.). (2005). *Alkohol och hälsa- en kunskapsöversikt om alkoholens positiva och negativa effekter på vår hälsa*. Rapport 2005:11. Stockholm: Statens Folkhälsöinstitutet.
Armstrong, E. (2003). *Conceiving risk, bearing responsibility. Fetal alcohol syndrome and the diagnosis of a moral disorder*. Baltimore, MD: The John Hopkins University Press.
Armstrong, E., & Abel, E. (2002). Fetal alcohol syndrome: The origins of a moral panic. *Alcohol and Alcoholism*, *35*(3), 276–282. doi:10.1093/alcalc/35.3.276
Bell, K. (2014). Science, policy and the rise of 'thirdhand smoke' as a public health issue. *Health, Risk & Society*, *16*(2), 154–170. doi:10.1080/13698575.2014.884214
Bell, K., McNaughton, D., & Salmon, A. (2009). Medicine, morality and mothering: Public health discourses on foetal alcohol exposure, smoking around children and childhood overnutrition. *Critical Public Health*, *19*(2), 155–170. doi:10.1080/09581590802385664
The Best Start Possible. (2009). *Advice for those planning or expecting a child, IS-1758*. Oslo: Sosial- og helsedirektoratet.
Cohen, S. (1972). *Folk devils and moral panics*. London: Routledge.
Daniels, C. (1993). *At women's expense: State power and the politics of foetal rights*. Cambridge, MA: Harvard University Press.
Den bedste start. (2009). Sundhedsstyrelsen. Retrieved June 24, 2012, from http://www.denbedstestart.dk/en.aspx
Douglas, M. (1992). *Risk and blame: Essays in cultural theory*. London: Routledge.
Douglas, M., & Wildavsky, A. (1982). *Risk and culture: An essay on the selection of environmental and technological dangers*. Berkeley: University of California Press.
Drabble, L. A., Poole, N., Magri, R., Tumwesigye, N. M., Li, Q., & Plant, M. (2011). Conceiving risk, divergent responses: Perspectives on the construction of risk of FASD in six countries. *Substance Use Misuse*, *46*(8), 943–958. doi:10.3109/10826084.2010.527419
Ewald, F. (2002). The return of descartes's malicious demon: An outline of a philosophy of precaution. In T. Baker & J. Simon (Eds.), *Embracing risk: The changing culture of risk and responsibility* (pp. 273–302). Chicago, IL: The University of Chicago Press.
Folkhälsöinstitutet. (2009). *Barnmorskans guide för samtal om alkohol* [Guide to midwives for discussing alcohol issues]. Växjö: Statens folkhälsoinstitut.
Furedi, F. (2002). *Paranoid parenting. Why ignoring the experts may be the best for your child*. Chicago, IL: Chicago Review Press.
Gavaghan, C. (2009). "You can't handle the truth": Medical paternalism and prenatal alcohol use. *Journal of Medical Ethics*, *35*, 300–303. doi:10.1136/jme.2008.028662

Golden, J. (2005). *Message in the bottle. The making of fetal alcohol syndrom.* Cambridge: Harvard University Press.

Göransson, M., & Magnusson, Å. (2005). Måttlig alkoholkonsumtion under graviditet [Moderate alcohol consumption during pregnancy]. In S. Andréasson & P. Allebeck (Eds.), *Alkohol och hälsa- en kunskapsöversikt om alkoholens positiva och negativa effekter på vår hälsa.* Rapport 2005:11. Stockholm: Statens Folkhälsöinstitutet.

Gray, R., Mukherjee, R. A. S., & Rutter, M. (2009). Alcohol consumption during pregnancy and its effects on neurodevelopment: What is known and what remains uncertain (for debate). *Addiction, 104*(8), 1270–1273. doi:10.1111/j.1360-0443.2008.02441.x

Hammer, R., & Inglin, S. (2014). 'I don't think it's risky, but…': Pregnant women's risk perceptions of maternal drinking and smoking. *Health, Risk & Society, 16*(1), 22–35. doi:10.1080/13698575.2013.863851

Healthy habits – before, during and after pregnancy. (2010). (1st English edition, translated from the 2nd Danish edition 2010). Copenhagen: The Danish National Board of Health and The Danish Committee for Health Education.

Hendersson, J., Gray, R., & Brocklehurst, P. (2007). Systematic review of effects of low-moderate prenatal alcohol exposure on pregnancy outcome. *International Journal of Obstetrics and Gynaeology, 114*(3), 243–252. doi:10.1111/j.1471-0528.2006.01163.x

Järvinen, M. (2012). A will to health? Drinking, risk and social class. *Health, Risk & Society, 14*(3), 241–256. doi:10.1080/13698575.2012.662632

Jyllands Posten. (2012, June 20). Skål, du er gravid.

Kaskutas, L. A. (1995). Interpretations of risk: The use of scientific information in the development of the alcohol warning lapbel policy. *The International Journal of the Addictions, 30*(12), 1519–1548.

Käypä hoito. (2012). The Finnish Medical Society Duodecim. Retrieved June 22, 2012, from http://www.kaypahoito.fi/web/kh/suositukset/suositus?id=hoi50028

Keane, H. (2013). Healthy adults and maternal bodies: Reformulations of gender in Australian alcohol guidelines. *Health Sociology Review, 22*(2), 151–161. doi:10.5172/hesr.2013.22.2.151

Kesmodel, U. (2006). Alkohol og evidens – om at læsa litteraturen [Alcohol and evidence – how to read the literature]. *Ugeskrift for Læger, 168*(12), 1214.

Kukla, R. (2010). The ethics and cultural politics of reproductive risk warnings: A case study of California's proposition 65. *Health, Risk & Society, 12*, 323–334.

Leppo, A. (2012). *Precarious pregnancies. Alcohol, drugs and the regulation of risks* (Publications of the Department of Social Research 2012: 3). Helsinki: Unigrafia.

Leppo, A., & Hecksher, D. (2011). The rise of the total abstinence model. Recommendations regarding alcoholuse during pregnancy in Finland and Denmark. *Nordic Studies on Alcohol and Drugs, 28*(1), 7–27. doi:10.2478/v10199-011-0002-7

Livsmedelsverket. (2008). Toxikologiska risker vid graviditet och amning – vetenskapligt underlag inför revideringen av livsmedelsverkets kostråd för gravida. Livsmedelsverket. Retrieved January 1, 2012, from http://www.slv.se/upload/dokument/mat/kostrad/gravida_ammande/toxikologiska_risker_graviditet_amning_2008.pdf

Livsmedelsverket. (2009). *Råd om bra mat för gravida – Handledning för mödrahälsovården* [Advice on food for pregnant women – Guidelines for maternity care]. Uppsala: Livsmedelsverket.

Lowe, P., & Lee, E. (2010). Advocating alcohol abstinence to pregnant women: Some observations about British policy. *Health Risk & Society, 12*(4), 301–311. doi:10.1080/13698571003789690

Lupton, D. (2011). 'The best thing for the baby': Mothers' concepts and experiences related to promoting their infants' health and development. *Health, Risk & Society, 13*(7–8), 637–651. doi:10.1080/13698575.2011.624179

Lupton, D. (2012). 'Precious cargo': Foetal subjects, risk and reproductive citizenship. *Critical Public Health, 22*(3), 329–340. doi:10.1080/09581596.2012.657612

O'Leary, C., & Bower, C. (2011). Guidelines for pregnancy: What's an acceptable risk and how is the evidence (finally) shaping up? *Drug and Alcohol Review, 31*(2), 170–183. doi:10.1111/j.1465-3362.2011.00331.x

O'Leary, C. M., Heuzenroeder, L., Elliot, E., & Bower, C. (2007). A review of policies on alcohol use during pregnancy in Australia and other English-speaking counries. *The Medical Journal of Australia, 186*, 466–471.

Oakley, A. (1989). Smoking in pregnancy: Smokescreen or risk factor? Toward a materialist analysis. *Sociology of Health and Illness, 11*(4), 311–335. doi:10.1111/1467-9566.ep11372513

Osimani, B. (2013). The precautionary principle in the pharmaceutical domain: A philosophical enquiry into probabilistic reasoning and risk aversion. *Health, Risk & Society*, *15*(2), 123–143. doi:10.1080/13698575.2013.771736

Plant, M. (1997). *Women and alcohol. Contemporary and historical perspectives*. New York, NY: Free Association Books.

Room, R. (2005). Fetal alcohol syndrome: A biography of a diagnosis. *The Lancet*, *365*(11), 1999–2000. doi:10.1016/S0140-6736(05)66681-0

Rothman, B. K. (1986). *The tentative pregnancy. Amniocentesis and the sexual politics of motherhood*. London: Pandora.

Rothman, B. K. (2014). Pregnancy, birth and risk: An introduction. *Health, Risk & Society*, *16*(1), 1–6. doi:10.1080/13698575.2013.876191

Scamell, M., & Stewart, M. (2014). Time, risk and midwife practice: The vaginal examination. *Health, Risk & Society*, *16*(1), 84–100. doi:10.1080/13698575.2013.874549

Scamell, M. A., & Alaszewski, A. (2012). Fateful moments and the categorisation of risk: Midwifery practice and the ever-narrowing window of normality during childbirth. *Health, Risk & Society*, *14*(2), 107–115. doi:10.1080/13698575.2012.661041

Sokol, R., Delaney-Black, V., & Nordstrom, B. (2003). Fetal alcohol spectrum disorder. *JAMA*, *290*, 2996–2999.

Sosiaali- ja terveysministeriö. (2007). *Seksuaali- ja lisääntymisterveyden edistäminen. Toimintaohjelma 2007–2011* [Promotion of sexual and reproductive health. Action programme 2007–2011]. Helsinki: Sosiaali- ja terveysministeriön julkaisuja 17.

Sosial- og helsedirektoratet. (2005a). *Alkohol og graviditet: Hva er farlig for fosteret? Hvordan forebygge og behandle? Rapport fra en ekspertgruppe*, IS-1284 [Alcohol and pregnancy. What are the risks for the fetus? How to prevent and treat? Report from the expert group]. Oslo: Author.

Sosial- og helsedirektoratet. (2005b). *Retningslinjer for svangerskapsomsorgen, IS-1179*. Oslo: A National Clinical Guideline for Antenatal Care.

Strandberg-Larsen, K., & Grønbæk, M. (2006). *Notat vedrørende alkohol og graviditet*. Copenhagen: Center for Alkoholforskning, Statens Institut for Folkesundhed. (Memorandum on alcohol and pregnancy for the Danish National Board of Health).

Sundhedsstyrelsen. (2009). *Anbefalinger for svangreomsorgen* [Recommendations for antenatal care]. København: Sundhedsstyrelsen.

Törrönen, J., & Tryggvesson, K. (2014). Alcohol, health and reproduction. *Critical Discourse Studies*. Advance online publication. doi:10.1080/17405904.2014.934386

Tryggvesson, K. (2005, May 30–June 3). *Campaigning against drinking during pregnancy – in the interest of whom?* Paper presented at the Annual Alcohol Epidemiology Symposium of the Kettil Bruun Society in 2005, Riverside, CA.

We're having a baby. (2009). Helsinki: Stakes

Zinn, J. O. (2009). The sociology of risk and uncertainty a response to Judith Green's is it time for the sociology of health to abandon risk. *Health, Risk & Society*, *11*(6), 509–526. doi:10.1080/13698570903329490

To what extent are women free to choose where to give birth? How discourses of risk, blame and responsibility influence birth place decisions

Kirstie Coxon[a], Jane Sandall[a] and Naomi J. Fulop[b]

[a]Division of Women's Health, Women's Health Academic Centre (King's Health Partners), King's College London, London, UK; [b]Department of Applied Health Research, University College London, London, UK

Over the past 50 years, two things have changed for women giving birth in high-income nations; birth has become much safer, and now takes place in hospital rather than at home. The extent to which these phenomena are related is a source of ongoing debate, but concern about high intervention rates in hospitals, and financial pressures on health care systems, have led governments, clinicians and groups representing women to support a return to birth in 'alternative' settings such as midwife-led birth centres or at home, particularly for well women with healthy pregnancies. Despite this, most women still plan to give birth in high-technology hospital labour wards. In this article, we draw on a longitudinal narrative study of pregnant women at three maternity services in England between October 2009 and November 2010. Our findings indicate that for many women, hospital birth with access to medical care remained the default option. When women planned hospital birth, they often conceptualised birth as medically risky, and did not raise concerns about overuse of birth interventions; instead, these were considered an essential form of rescue from the uncertainties of birth. Those who planned birth in alternative settings also emphasised their intention, and obligation, to seek medical care if necessary. Using sociocultural theories of risk to focus our analysis, we argue that planning place of birth is mediated by cultural and historical associations between birth and safety, and further influenced by prominent contemporary narratives of risk, blame and the responsibility. We conclude that even with high-level support for 'alternative' settings for birth, these discourses constrain women's decisions, and effectively limit opportunities for planning birth in settings other than hospital labour wards. Our contention is that a combination of cultural and social factors helps explain the continued high uptake of hospital obstetric unit birth, and that for this to change, birth in alternative settings would need to be positioned as a culturally normative and acceptable practice.

Introduction

Planning where to give birth is arguably one of the most important decisions made during pregnancy, yet it is often taken for granted that birth takes place in hospital. Recent history shows that this remains the case despite almost 50 years of challenges to 'technological' birth by lay groups, feminist scholars and other maternity activists. These groups have

Box 1. Terms used to denote different birth facilities or settings.

OU – Obstetric Unit ('labour ward'): Provides 24 hour routine and emergency maternity care, with access to NICU; staffed by midwives, obstetricians and other specialists.
Ninety-three per cent of births in England take place in obstetric units.
AMU – Alongside Midwifery Unit ('birth centre' or 'snoezelen room') – Maternity unit staffed and led by midwives, co-located on site of an obstetric unit but organisationally separate. No epidural or surgical services.
Three per cent of births in England take place in AMUs.
FMU – Freestanding Midwifery Unit ('birth centre'). Maternity unit on a separate, community site, not based in a tertiary hospital. Staffed by midwives, no epidural or surgical services.
Two per cent of births in England take place in FMUs.
Home birth – birth in woman's own home, supported by a midwife (legal and provided free of charge through NHS care in the United Kingdom).
Around three per cent of births in England take place at home.

Source for definitions: Rowe (2011).
Source for proportion of births in each setting: HCC (2008).

long argued that hospital birth, with its reliance on surveillance medicine, high-technology equipment and adherence to protocol-led care, changes birth from a positive, life-affirming rite of passage to a dehumanised, mechanistic process. It is now well established that when healthy women with low-risk pregnancies give birth in traditional hospital labour wards (or obstetric units 'OUs' – see Box 1 for categorisation of the types of facilities available to women), they are more likely to experience interventions, surgical birth and their sequelae; what then accounts for the continued popularity of the 'hospital' birth model?

Drawing on empirical narrative research with pregnant women in England, in this article, we explore women's experiences of deciding where to give birth. Our starting point is an acknowledgement that such decisions are taken under conditions of uncertainty, when the outcome is unknown. By drawing on sociocultural concepts of risk, we begin to tease apart the subtle impact brought to bear on these decisions by discourses of risk, blame and responsibility. We argue that beliefs and assumptions about birth risk are deeply ingrained, reflect varying perceptions of who is to blame if things go wrong and incorporate differing views of both nature and technology in relation to birth. We start the article with a discussion of existing literature in relation to birth place preference, we then review wider public debates about how the relationship between medical technology and nature influences constructions of birth as 'safe', 'risky' or 'uncertain', before presenting findings from our empirical research.

Risk, choice and place of birth

In England, there has been high-level policy support for choice of place of birth for two decades (Department of Health 1993, 2007), yet giving birth in settings other than a hospital OU (or 'labour ward') remains unusual. Over the past two decades, the proportion of home births in England has remained virtually static at around 2.5%, although national data (HCC 2008) shows that a further 5% of women now give birth in alongside or freestanding midwifery units (AMUs or FMUs – see Box 1).

Previous studies of birth place decisions consistently show that hospital birth is associated with safety for many women (Houghton *et al.* 2008, Pitchforth *et al.* 2008,

2009). Birth place preferences are also thought to be influenced by socio-economic status (Nelson 1983, Davis-Floyd 1990, 1992, Zadoroznyj 1999), by access to private or publicly funded models of care (Liamputtong 2005, Murray and Elston 2005), by moral considerations (Viisainen 2000) and by cultural, religious and ethnic allegiances (Donner 2003).

Scholars have also argued that women associate different risks with different settings for birth (for example, Davis-Floyd 1990, 1992, Abel and Kearns 1991, Devries *et al.* 2001, Bryant *et al.* 2007). Women who prefer home birth are usually described as being concerned about risks imposed *on* 'natural' birth *by* birth in a hospital, and by separation from their families (e.g. Abel and Kearns 1991, Davis-Floyd 1992, Edwards 2005, Cheyney 2008). In contrast, women who prefer hospital birth are thought to be concerned about the risks and uncertainties *of* 'natural' birth, preferring to 'stay in control' and seeing hospital medical technology as a means of reducing risk by securing a clinically 'clean' and 'safe' birth, with access to anaesthetic pain relief during labour (Davis-Floyd 1994, Bryant *et al.* 2007). The assumption that women's birth place decisions are polarised between preference for either 'natural' or 'medical' birth has rested largely unchallenged in the sociological literature since the early 1970s, and this dichotomy increasingly fails to capture the nuances of women's experiences, or the breadth of contextual influences upon their decisions (Coxon 2012). The polarisation of 'natural' vs. 'technological' perspectives of birth also reflects a debate central to risk theory identified by Zinn (2008, p. 439), which is the attempt to contrast the relative merits of 'objective' or 'rational' knowledge (associated with an 'expert'-led technological knowledge) with 'non-rational strategies' informed by personal experiences, beliefs and socially mediated knowledge such as folk-wisdom or 'old wives' tales'. Zinn (2008) argues that in practice, individual decision-making relies on strategies which are 'in between' these extremes, leading to decisions which not only draw upon objective knowledge, but are also infused with intuition, trust and emotion.

In recent decades, 'home-like' settings in maternity hospitals have been provided in many high-income countries. 'Alongside midwife-led units' or 'birth centres' provide low-technology midwife-led care to carefully screened healthy women whose pregnancies are categorised as 'low-risk' (Hodnett *et al.* 2010), with the additional 'safety net' of easy access to high-technology care, should this be required. Such units might be considered an attempt by hospital institutions to address exactly this need to manage the uncertainty of birth with an 'in-between' setting, both humane and home-like but with rapid access to high-tech facilities. In England, the provision of AMUs in maternity hospitals has expanded rapidly in recent years (Redshaw *et al.* 2011), and these increasingly appear to be the preferred solution to the 'problem' of providing women with both choice *and* safe, high-quality, individualised maternity care.

Birth place decisions in the United Kingdom: is birth safe or risky?

Childbirth in the United Kingdom is increasingly considered to be 'safe', at least relative to low-income countries without health infrastructure or access to trained and qualified birth attendants. However, a combination of higher maternal age, an ethnically diverse population, rising caesarean rates and increasing levels of obesity and chronic disease, such as diabetes, mean that more pregnancies are medically complex, and demand for tertiary-level, critical and intensive care in maternity services is increasing (RCOG 2013).

Despite these public health challenges, women and babies in England are demonstrably safer during birth than was once the case, yet birth is still understood and, to some extent, experienced as 'risky' or potentially so. In the context of welfare, Taylor-Gooby (2000, p. 4) described anxiety about risk where evidence suggests improved health, wealth and security as 'timid prosperity', occurring where 'concern [about risk] is pervasive although vulnerability is concentrated among the weakest groups in an increasingly unequal society'. In relation to birth, this seems to be the case; women who do not have universal access to high-quality maternity care bear much of the burden of poor outcomes, but those in more affluent settings remain highly sensitised to the presumed risks of birth. In common with Giddens (1991) and Beck (1992), Taylor-Gooby considers this to be evidence of risk reflexivity, which occurs as a consequence of well-educated, affluent populations developing 'more critical attitudes to received wisdom and to professional expertise' (2000, p. 10).

Despite the critical and reflexive responses to expert notions of risk that these theories anticipate, there remains an enduring public acceptance that births ought to take place in hospital OUs, particularly for first babies (Topliss 1970, Cunningham 1993, Barber et al. 2006). Contemporary discourses of parenthood, examples of which are found in media debates on parenting, advertising targeted at parents, parenting magazines and advice provided by professionals involved in supporting parents and parents-to-be, ensure parents are made aware that they must be seen to be responsible, effective 'risk managers' in relation to birth, upbringing and infant feeding (Green 1999, Lee 2008, Scamell 2011, Scamell and Alaszewski 2012). Parents-to-be, particularly pregnant women, are also required to demonstrate moral, physical and emotional 'fitness' for pregnancy and beyond (Marshall and Woollett 2000, Mansfield 2008, Nash 2011). Green (1999, p. 29) has also charted increasing societal unwillingness to describe or accept deaths as 'accidental', and argues that deaths once considered as misfortunes have been re-categorised as an outcome of mismanaged risk, something that 'should never have happened in the first place' (2007, p. 35). That this was the case in relation to place of birth by the turn of the 1960s can be inferred from the following (anonymous) editorial comment in the Lancet: 'Good antenatal care and safe delivery in a hospital fully equipped and staffed to deal with any emergency can prevent family tragedies once thought to be unavoidable' (Lancet 1963, p. 1208, emphasis added).

The view that birth in hospital is essential to prevent death is the product of a powerful historical discourse, and one which has been reiterated by sources perceived as authoritative, with international reach and influence.

Sociocultural theories of risk, blame and normality

The belief that scientific or technological advances create dangers as well as solutions is also part of the 'risk society' thesis (Giddens 1991, Beck 1992). Beck, in particular, argues that reflexive anxiety about risk is a consequence of global technological advances, because the risks these carry are beyond the control of government or the democratic will of individuals or nations. A decade earlier, Douglas and Wildavsky (1982) had also tried to tackle the paradoxical increase in risk anxiety which seemed to accompany improved levels of security and well-being. In Risk and Culture, Douglas and Wildavsky (1982) examined why it might be that an increasingly affluent US population, apparently benefitting from cheap nuclear energy and improved living standards, developed an increasing aversion to the technological and environmental risks of nuclear power. They concluded that 'technological' risks, rather than necessarily being 'objectively real' or 'measurable', are better understood as having been 'selected' from an array of potential hazards, to support and validate a particular political perspective (for example, being pro-nature, and opposed to pollution, or other impacts of scientific or technological activity on the environment). A further insight, drawn from Douglas' earlier anthropological studies (Douglas 1966, 1970), was that the opportunity to allocate blame is central to the selection of risks: 'Blameworthiness takes over at the point where the line of normality is drawn. Each culture rests upon its own ideas of what ought to be normal or natural. If a death is held to be normal, no-one is blamed' (Douglas and Wildavsky 1982, p. 35).

In this article, we examine the extent to which these sociocultural approaches to risk might enhance our understanding of contemporary birth place decisions. As we have argued, for 'natural birth' proponents, birth at home or in a non-OU setting minimises 'unnecessary intervention', and provides the best opportunity for labour and birth to be a fulfilling, life-enhancing experience, to assist with the transition to parenthood and relationship formation between mother and child (Kitzinger 2005, Fahy *et al.* 2008) and increasingly, though to a lesser extent, father and child (Miller 2011). Detractors argue that whilst birth without obstetricians to hand may be safe for many, it is unsafe for a few, or at least associated with untenable pain, and difficulty in predicting who will benefit and who will suffer makes an OU the 'rational', common-sense answer. The increasing costs of insuring obstetric and maternity care, particularly in relation to lifelong claims for damage and disability in infants, provide a further strand to this complex situation. As well as potential medical and obstetric risks, birth carries litigation and reputational risks for professionals. This leads to 'litigation–based practice' (Dahlen and Homer 2013, p. 168), where birth risks are managed through adherence to (and sponsoring women's compliance with) 'active management' protocols and procedures, to reduce professional and organisational exposure to medico-legal risk.

Birth may then be constructed as both safe and potentially risky, for women, babies and clinicians, and choosing home, or birth in a midwife-led setting over a traditional OU birth might either increase or decrease perceptions of different types of risk, depending on the perspective adopted. Comparative epidemiology and public health evidence shows that some birth risk is objectively present, although rare, but qualitative studies reveal that women and partners' risk perceptions are often subjectively distorted beyond the level of 'actual' threat (Houghton *et al.* 2008). It is likely that the heightened perception of risk goes some way towards explaining women's birth place preferences, but this alone fails to account for why some women come to adopt strong opposition to birth in hospital OUs, whilst others positively opt for this. The research described in this paper arose from a need to understand better what accounts for birth place preferences, particularly the continued uptake of hospital OUs, in a context where alternative settings, whilst not always immediate or accessible, are freely provided and actively promoted, yet remain under-used.

Method

Much research into this subject has relied on single interviews, often conducted retro-spectively, after birth has taken place. This has the effect of producing results based on women's sense-making of their birth experiences, sometimes many years after the event. This research used a prospective, longitudinal narrative interview design in order to provide a contemporaneous account of women's views and beliefs about place of birth, and to identify any changes which occurred over the course of pregnancy. We used a narrative methodology to prompt unguided accounts, through the use of a single 'narra-tive-eliciting' question at the beginning of each interview, which invited participants to discuss where they planned to give birth, and any events or experiences which contributed to this. In shorter 'end of pregnancy' interviews, we asked women to comment on their experiences since the first interview, and explored whether their views or birth place intentions had altered in the interim.

We decided to use the narrative method as a means of inviting accounts without 'framing' the study in terms of risk or safety, which, as Henwood *et al.* (2010) note, can mean that researchers' *a priori* assumptions about risk form the basis of the investigation, rather than allowing new or different perspectives to emerge. Our approach was informed by Wengraf's (2001) biographical-narrative interpretative methodology, and we adopted Riessman's analytical methods for exploring how accounts are ordered and structured (Riessman 2008), and assessing the moral positioning of the self as a protagonist within the account (Bury 2001, Ehrich 2003). Ethical approval was granted by a National Health Service (NHS) research ethics committee [09/H0808/45].

Fieldwork was undertaken between October 2009 and November 2010 at three maternity services in England. The sites included inner city and semi-rural locations with different geographies and transfer time scenarios. Birth place options varied between the sites, but women had access to home birth (all sites), FMUs (one site), AMUs (two sites) and OUs (all sites). The proportion of births taking place in AMU, FMU or at home in these sites ranged from 6.7% to 18.5%, and was near or above the average for England (7%) at the time the fieldwork was undertaken (HCC 2008).

We recruited a diverse sample (Patton 2002) in order to explore the extent to which accounts of birth place risk and safety varied amongst respondents with different parity, birth experiences, socio-economic, cultural and ethnic backgrounds. Initial recruitment yielded a relatively homogenous sample, but following ethical approval of a substantial amendment to the original protocol, store vouchers for £20 were provided to participants in recognition of the time contributed to the research. The final sample included 41 women recruited at antenatal clinics or through interpreters (birth partners were also recruited, but this paper presents only findings from interviews with pregnant women). Participants were aged 19–42, from various ethnic backgrounds, five of whom required an interpreter to participate. Interviewees held a range of qualifications, and employment status varied. Just under half were expecting their first baby (44%), reflecting the national average (ONS 2009). Married, cohabiting and single women took part. Overall, respondents were slightly older and held higher qualifications than is the case in the maternal population (when compared with national and regional data sets) but there was diversity in terms of employment, spoken English, education and ethnicity.

Most initial interviews took place between 12 and 24 weeks of pregnancy at women's homes, and a small number were conducted by telephone, where this was the woman's preference. Interviews lasted between 30 and 75 minutes, but were usually about an hour long. Short follow-up telephone interviews were carried out in the last month of pregnancy. All interviews were conducted by the same researcher [Kirstie Coxon]. Altogether, 82 interviews were undertaken, with no loss to follow-up.

Interviews were digitally recorded and transcribed, with the exception of three participants who preferred not to be audio-recorded; these interviews were documented in contemporaneous field notes. Interview transcripts and field notes were entered into N-Vivo 8 (N-Vivo 8 QSR International Pty Ltd.) and initially analysed using thematic narrative analysis (Riessman 2008). This approach uses a coding process similar to grounded theory method, but with some key differences; in narrative thematic analyses, context is retained, text is interpreted in relation to each woman's overall 'story', and interviewer prompts and questions, or other interruptions, are retained and considered part of the co-constructed interview discourse.

Antenatal data analyses were also 'future-blind', meaning that they were undertaken before the outcome of the pregnancy and actual place of birth were known. In narrative analysis, the 'outcome' of the story is understood to change how the events are interpreted by the teller and by the listener, so 'future-blind' analysis helped identify women's pre-birth beliefs, concerns and aspirations before these were altered by the course of events. Disconfirming or theoretically ambiguous data were discussed with co-authors [Jane Sandall and Naomi Fulop], peer researchers and service user groups to clarify and make sense of the issues that these raised.

Findings

In this article, we draw on data from the interviews to examine how women made sense of birth risk and the uncertainties they faced during pregnancy, and related these factors to their planned place of birth. From a clinical perspective, three quarters of participants (30 out of 41) had healthy pregnancies, making them eligible for birth in a full range of possible settings (home birth, FMU, AMU or OU). The remainder (11 out of 41) had a risk factor which meant they either required further assessment, or would routinely be advised to give birth in a hospital OU according to existing English National Institute of Health and Care Excellence (NICE) guidance (NCCWCH 2007). The reason for recruiting women with both clinically healthy pregnancies and with risk factors present was to explore the 'fit' between messages received from health professionals or others about the riskiness or otherwise of their pregnancies and women's own expectations of birth risk.

As others (Lee *et al.* 2012) have also found, women's perspectives could differ markedly from clinical risk assessments. Some felt they could safely give birth at home despite having clinical risk factors which meant that hospital OU birth would be recommended. This viewpoint was however relatively unusual; it was far more often the case that women were healthy and had 'low-risk' pregnancies, but could not countenance giving birth anywhere other than hospital OUs. There was also a clear difference in experience between women expecting their first babies, and those who had given birth before; in first pregnancies, women were more open to the idea of birth in different settings, but those expecting second or subsequent babies usually planned hospital OU births. For this reason, findings are presented separately for each group.

Where extracts from interviews are presented in this paper, pseudonyms are used and broad contextual information is provided, although identifying details have been removed. In interviewee quotes, pauses of up to three seconds are denoted by an ellipse within square brackets [...]. Non-bracketed ellipses indicate that some text has been removed, usually to shorten the quote, but the sequence of the narrative is unaltered.

Prioritising 'medical' risks of birth: planning birth in a hospital obstetric unit

When women preferred to give birth in hospital OUs, their accounts often presented birth as medically risky or subject to danger. Most women in the sample (25 out of 41) planned to give birth in hospital OUs by the final month of pregnancy. Of these, 11 had risk factors which meant that OU would be recommended for birth, but 14 had healthy pregnancies, and it is on this group that we focus here, given that they could all have chosen home birth (because this is available in all the areas where recruitment took place) and most had access to either AMU or FMUs too. Seven were expecting their first baby, and seven were planning their second or subsequent birth.

Accounts from women expecting their first babies

When women planned to have their first baby in hospital OUs, it was often because they feared something might go wrong, or had received advice from close family to give birth in hospital. Kath described a discussion in her midwife 'booking' appointment in early pregnancy as follows:

> I was really surprised actually because [...] I'm 38 and ... I'm not the world's fittest person ... and I was convinced that I was going to be some high-risk kind of, oh my gosh, you can't step out of [a hospital labour ward]. So I was quite surprised when I came out low-risk, and [the midwife] said 'Do you want a home birth?' (Kath, expecting first baby, healthy pregnancy, planned OU birth)

Kath's concerns related to overall age and general fitness, and these respond to existing discourse of being 'fit' to give birth (Mansfield 2008, Nash 2011). Other women were sceptical about the likelihood of an out-of-hospital birth being safe for themselves or their babies because of their family histories. Laura had a healthy pregnancy and was expecting her first baby, but thought her relatives' experiences of birth might affect her own labour:

> In deciding where to have the baby, I guess I was pretty determined I'd have it in hospital [OU]. Both my sister and my mother had problems during birth, I was born by emergency caesarean and my sister had an emergency caesarean with her first child, and then an elective caesarean for her second, so it made sense given the experiences of people close to me that I'd like to be somewhere with good medical care on hand, if something goes wrong. (Laura, expecting first baby, healthy pregnancy, planned OU birth)

Donna's general medical practitioner (GP) advised her to avoid going to her local FMU with her first baby, and his concerns chimed with her own risk perceptions:

> I said, 'Look, don't worry, I'm not going anywhere there's no doctors.' And he said, 'Yes, I'm just saying, you know, because you know the chances are ... It's a 40 minute journey [referring to transfer to OU during labour]. Do you want to risk that?' No! [Laughs] But yeah, that's all he really said, but he was right...I'm not risking that, I'm not risking the baby's life or my life. So ... you know, it's just eliminating all the risks as much as you possibly can. (Donna, first baby, healthy pregnancy, planned OU birth)

In their narratives, Kath and Laura stopped short of making the 'risks' of birth explicit; instead, they alluded to the need for a hospital labour ward and access to emergency caesareans. Donna, on the other hand, was clear that she wouldn't risk 'the baby's life or my life' by giving birth in a place without doctors. Referring to the 'worst-case scenario' in this way heightened the dramatic effect of the statement, and communicated Donna's sense of anxiety about birth. In each of these accounts, 'hospital' was used as a short-hand to refer to obstetric medical care and a sense of protection from risk; 'alternatives' were not mentioned, and women did not anticipate having water births or similar 'natural birth' experiences in hospital OUs. The hospital itself was associated with safety and reassurance; later in her interview, Kath described a major teaching hospital in the following terms: 'But yeah, it is that kind of, yeah. I've fallen for the propaganda, it's that lovely big sign outside, which says "comfort". Yeah, it feels really comforting'.

Accounts from women expecting their second or subsequent baby

Women expecting their second or subsequent babies often have had previous normal births themselves, but were still influenced by the experiences of others close to them. Patsy's account illustrated this well, and she linked her decision to give birth in hospital OU, despite liking the idea of the facilities in FMU or AMU settings, to a sibling's experience of stillbirth.

> My brother had … well his wife had a baby at home and the baby died … and I think that affects … that sort of affects the family for a long time, you know, anyone in the family who was involved with that or remembers that, you can't, [home birth is] just a no-no for us. (Patsy, multiparous, healthy pregnancy and straightforward obstetric history, planned OU birth)

Later in the interview, Patsy mentioned that her mother also had a child born with a disability at home. The clustering of infant death or disability within families may reflect socio-economic inequities or genetic conditions, but the impact is passed down through generations, and to plan a home birth could be construed as insensitive to affected family members, and implicitly disrespectful towards shared family memories.

For women born in countries other than the United Kingdom, family practices were also important, and these reflected the national context of birth in both developing and high-income countries. Alexandria's family lived in Africa and although she had a healthy pregnancy and straightforward obstetric history, she was insistent that she should go to hospital OU to give birth.

> Well basically I think it's just what I've known. That's what my mother did, all my family members have had their babies in the hospital, and I just think it's a safer place, in case of any kind of emergency it's better to be at the hospital where there's a doctor close by.
> …I think it's culture as well, for me. It's just where we're from. You only have a baby at home if you can't make it to the hospital, and even when that happens people are […] almost ashamed to say. They'll still say, 'Oh yeah, we went to the hospital.'

Preference for hospital OU was also found amongst families from European countries where hospital OU is the only birth option available. Hannah described a conversation with her birth partner, who had asked whether she wanted to give birth at home:

> I just thought, what? What a strange thing to ask. Because for me, being [from a Nordic country], when you want to have babies, you go to the hospital, just like if you want to have an operation you go to hospital! (Hannah, multiparous, healthy pregnancy, planned OU birth)

Amongst women who had previously given birth, the sense that birth *ought* to take place in hospital emerged through tacit knowledge or received wisdom, which had been absorbed through family life and inter-generational life histories, but was also representative of national cultural discourses and normative practice. These inherited ideas and traditions might feasibly be brought into question by the events of women's own previous labours, or by different approaches in the new, host country, but it seemed to be more often the case that beliefs learned through upbringing and family practices endured.

Women expecting their first babies did not have past labour to draw upon, and amongst this group, perceived medical-obstetric risks of birth were an important basis for preferring hospital birth, but these rationalities supplemented an existing canon of expectations in relation to place of birth.

Conceptualising the 'risks' of hospital obstetric unit birth

Regardless of whether or not they had given birth before, women who planned to give birth in hospital OU discussed their need to determine which NHS hospital was most likely to provide them with the best care. The context of media is relevant here; health care is frequently subject to debate in the UK mass media, and headlines reflect the national characteristic of passionate support for universal NHS health care and equally passionate assertions that the population is being failed by an underfunded or overly bureaucratic health system. Although NHS heath care is free, and only a tiny proportion (0.5%) of women have private obstetric or midwifery care, private in vitro fertilisation (IVF) clinics often provide services to the NHS, and so women may encounter private provision at this time. Serena had experienced assisted conception, and implicitly felt that a more private-*like* setting might have more chance of success:

> I mean I must admit when I went to [NHS obstetric hospital 1] to do the [fertility] programme, the offices were very kind of [...] very basic, quite [...] claustrophobic, you know, whereas [at NHS obstetric hospital 2] it was a new centre that they had, and even just the images on the wall, it had a feeling of like this is as if it's a private [...] you're walking into some kind of private unit. And not to say that [NHS obstetric hospital 1] couldn't have [achieved a successful pregnancy], but it gave you that feeling of not sitting down a corridor squashed together, everyone can hear what you're saying, it was very much [...] the way they presented themselves and the way the new unit, it felt like a new unit that they would have the better facilities. (Serena, first baby, healthy pregnancy, planned OU birth)

The need to avoid being 'squashed together' in 'busy' units conveys one of the perceived risks of NHS care. Hospitals were sometimes envisaged to be crowded, or chaotic, and there was a sense that women needed to compete for attention, and might even be overlooked:

> I just know how easily mistakes are made, and it worries me, that I'm putting my faith and the life of my child in a [...] in an overrun crowded hospital full of people giving birth [...] yes, does make me a bit nervous. But [...] we'll see. (Annette, first baby, healthy pregnancy, planned OU birth)

Others were also concerned about exposure to other people's physical or social conditions:

> You're more at risk because you're with people, you're surrounded by ... however many, 20 beds or something, and ... you know, another 40 couples that are having their babies and you don't know their health. And so disease, not disease but you know, things do spread. (Serena, expecting first baby, healthy pregnancy, planned OU birth)

In these accounts, OUs in hospital are privileged as sites of safety and protection because emergency care is available if '*something goes wrong*', but this needs to be balanced against some potential risks of being in hospital. These include exposure to overcrowding, errors and physical or social 'pollution', a term used here in the sense described by

Douglas and Wildavsky as 'a contagious state, harmful, caused by outside intervention' which 'carries the idea of a moral defect' (1982, pp. 36–37).

Although women were worried that maternity care might be anonymous, or error-prone, what is absent from these accounts is concern about high rates of intervention in maternity care. Inch (1982, p. 244) and others have conceptualised the 'cascade of intervention', a scenario where one birth intervention (such as induction, or augmentation of labour) almost inevitably leads to another, incrementally increasing the likelihood of an instrumental or surgical birth at each stage and reducing the chances that the woman will have a 'natural' birth. Surgical births and their clinical sequelae (haemorrhage, pain, infection) are then linked with further deleterious effects such as difficulties breastfeeding or 'bonding' with babies, and slow recovery from the medical-surgical birth experience. Given that this discourse of intervention as 'risky' to natural birth has been successfully expounded for 30 years and more, and is part of antenatal teaching, it might be expected that women would consider this to be problematic. However, this rarely featured in the narrative accounts of women who planned to give birth in hospital OUs. Instead, they positioned surgical interventions such as caesarean section as life-saving moments of rescue, to be adopted quickly if the clinical situation suggested they may be required. Laura's comment during an 'end of pregnancy' interview conveyed her sense of needing to 'try' for a 'natural' birth, but with recourse to surgery being part of that intention:

> We just won't let labour go on that long – if things aren't progressing, we'll ask for a caesarean section...I've done everything I can to be fit and healthy. I've done NCT [National Childbirth Trust[1]] – very helpful apart from they're a bit mad, and you have to take it with a pinch of salt. They are *very* pro- 'active birth' and anti-drug. (Laura, first baby, healthy pregnancy, planned OU birth; sister and mother had emergency caesareans)

In this extract, Laura discusses having worked hard to stay fit and healthy, and attending NCT birth preparation classes, both of which indicate self-presentation as a responsible, 'fit' parent-to-be. In England, most maternity hospitals offer birth preparation classes, but these are sometimes over-subscribed and women may opt for NCT classes, for which there is usually a charge. Not all women attend birth preparation classes, and a relatively small proportion access NCT classes. Laura's reflection on what she perceived as the NCT 'ethos', and her willingness to request a caesarean section, suggests that to some extent, she wished to distance herself from, or at least to challenge the authenticity of, a 'pro-"active birth" and anti-drug' ethos, allowing her to retain the option of technological care during birth.

Prioritising the 'iatrogenic' risks of birth interventions and preference for AMU, FMU or home birth

So far, we have discussed findings related to views and perspectives of women who planned to give birth in hospital OU, and this group included women expecting their first or subsequent babies, with and without clinical 'risk factors'. The rest of the sample (16 out of 41) planned to give birth either at home, in FMUs or in AMUs. As mentioned earlier, women expecting their first baby made up most of this group (10 out of 16), and almost all (15 out of 16) who wanted to give birth in a non-hospital setting had healthy pregnancies and straightforward obstetric histories.

In their accounts, these women referred to medical interventions during labour, and, as others have documented (Edwards 2005, Cheyney 2008), women who opted for non-OU births often intended to use non-pharmacological methods of pain relief, and to exert control over their birth, over the decisions made in labour, over the ambiance of the setting and presence of others in the birth environment. Marylin explained why she planned to give birth in an FMU as follows:

> I just really don't want to give birth in hospital [OU]. I don't like the environment very much and I prefer it to be kind of more natural, and without intervention as much as possible. So hence why I prefer to go to the [FMU] because it's kind of more natural and they kind of leave you to it, I don't really want epidurals or anything like that, I just want to kind of keep active throughout and [...] and do it all that way. (Marylin, expecting first baby, planned FMU birth)

She also compared her own hopes with her friend's induced labour, to explain why she wanted to avoid a 'more forced on you' birth:

> ...a close friend has given birth in hospital [OU] because she had to be induced, and the whole procedure [...] it just seems kind of more forced on you and more [...] scary, rather than just doing it at your own pace and dealing with it and the pain and everything that's happening at that time yourself. So ideally I'd stay [home] as long as possible and then go to the FMU.

Alison also sought control over her birth environment, having seen some conflicting accounts of hospital OU environments, particularly postnatal wards, on internet discussion fora:

> ...you've got control over your environment, you can decide what position you're in, whether you need something to eat or a bath or a scented candle or, you know, you might want none of those things, you might have time for none of those things... And being somewhere that is familiar and safe and happy and that is not intruded on by other people and their various dramas, positive or negative. And where you can control the cleanliness and the food and anything else, and you can go to your own bed afterwards and ... yes. It just feels to me some ... more comfortable. (Alison, expecting first baby, healthy pregnancy, planned home birth)

Hilary planned a home birth from the beginning of her pregnancy:

> ... I've kind of thought ... that it's worth aiming for the best-case [scenario] of being at home, and doing ... I mean the things that I've either started doing or been thinking about doing have been pregnancy yoga, which is much more about kind of relaxation techniques and breathing than it is about, I think, flexibility or normal yoga as we would think of it. And I've been thinking about getting a doula [paid birthing companion] as well – again, because I've heard quite good things about them through internet and through my own research... (Hilary, expecting first baby, healthy pregnancy, planned home birth)

In these accounts, the importance of relaxing in a private environment with known carers, having 'control' during labour, using alternatives to pharmacological pain relief were all evident; the 'risks' posed by hospital to natural birth, particularly the interventive approach associated with hospital OUs, were central to women's decisions to birth else-where. However, the medico-obstetric risks of birth, and concerns about safety, which were such an important feature of the narratives discussed earlier, were barely mentioned. Other 'risks' of hospital birth such as the busy environment and loss of privacy at a vulnerable time were also part of these narratives, but were cited as a reason for avoiding hospital OU, rather than something which has to be borne in order to secure the medical safety of specialist obstetric care.

Discussion

In this research, we sought not only to explore birth place decisions generally, but also to provide a contemporary account of preference for hospital OU care. We believe that our findings offer a more nuanced account of birth place preferences than that provided by the view that women's heightened anxiety about birth risks is sufficient to explain OU preference. This has implications for continued use of a 'polarisation' argument, whereby 'natural' and 'technological' views of birth are seen as being in opposition to each other, and as providing an explanatory framework for birth place decisions. Rather than choosing one stance over another, it seemed that women's responses were shaped by numerous discourses. These originated in family histories and childhood, incorporated national traditions of public health, and, for families who have moved to the United Kingdom in recent generations, the influence of home nation provider model of care seemed more powerful than the host nation's approach. These factors contributed to the immediate cultural milieux of interviewees, which was influenced by close family birth stories, as well as national cultural identities.

Previous studies on this topic have also recognised that although the rationale for providing alternatives to hospital OU may be to enhance access to 'natural' or 'low-technology' birth, women in fact seek control over birth in diverse ways. Authors have argued that some women eschew technology and embrace a 'natural', social or holistic approach (Garcia *et al.* 1990, Davis-Floyd and Sargent 1997, Viisainen 2000, 2001, Edwards 2005), whilst others suggest that sense of control is enhanced through 'technological' birth and 'choosing' medical interventions such as epidural anaesthesia or caesarean section (see Davis-Floyd 1990, 1994, Donner 2003, Bryant *et al.* 2007). Existing interpretative research on birth place decisions also suggests that women planning non-OU births still speak of the 'safety net' that specialist or acute care provides (Cheyney 2008, Pitchforth *et al.* 2008), although whether this is because women are mindful of 'medical-obstetric' risks of birth when planning a 'natural' non-OU birth, or concerned with the need to present themselves as moral, responsible, rational and 'fit' parents-to-be (Marshall and Woollett 2000, Viisainen 2001, Nash 2011) remains uncertain.

Using an analytic approach which incorporated ideas of sociocultural risk 'selection' led to a more detailed identification of individual birth risk perspectives. The narrative method was valuable in this endeavour, because it provided an opportunity to compare accounts, and consider which issues were neglected, as well as which were privileged or prioritised. The importance of safety from risk or harm was evident amongst narrative accounts of women who planned hospital OU birth, and this was often built on foundations already well established in family histories, so that the setting selected chimed best with what women already expected of birth, and of themselves during birth; over the course of time, cultural discourses had further attenuated women's sensitivity to and awareness of the 'medical' risks of birth. The 'problem' of medical intervention was therefore not recognised as such – instead, interventions were cast as an essential 'rescue' from the hazards or uncertainties of birth. This sits well with work by Zinn (2008, p. 445) and others (Taylor-Gooby 2000, Brown *et al.* 2011), which suggests that individuals seek to establish trust in institutions as a strategy for managing uncertainty. Zinn argues that 'stable institutions', established on the basis of dependable rules and protocols, might be viewed as a source of trust and security (2008, p. 448). As Scamell and Alaszewski (2012) point out, childbirth can be considered a 'fateful moment' in the sense outlined by Giddens (1991); a time when 'people might choose to have recourse to more traditional authorities' (p. 142). When maternity hospitals are thought of as sites of medical safety, it makes sense that women anticipate that these are the 'best' place for birth, even when adverse media coverage and an inquiry-based, 'name and shame' culture might reasonably be expected to unsettle this view. This may also help to explain why, when women planned hospital OU birth, the 'risks' that they discussed were not that they might experience iatrogenic complications, but instead included propensity for error, overcrowding and exposure to others' misfortunes, which threatened their view of hospital as a benevolent or stable institution.

The need to seek sanctuary during birth, coupled with a belief system that is sensitised to messages of riskiness and potential tragedy, might be sufficient to ensure women give birth in hospital OUs, but to this is added a strong societal expectation that parents take steps to actively present themselves as responsible and to be seen 'to do the right thing' in terms of self-education and preparation, which for many, includes planning to give birth in a hospital OU.

Whilst this was a prevailing perspective amongst interviewees, others had of course taken a different stance, and once again, risk selection helped to highlight some of the reasons for this. The principal feature of narratives which favoured non-OU birth 'alternatives' (home, FMU and AMU birth) was that the facilities and presentation of settings, and the extent to which one would be given privacy, dignity and individualised caregiver support, were considered very important. Here, the hospital OU was no longer an obvious safe haven, but instead characterised as a monolith, resistant to individualised needs and concerns, and where strict adherence to protocol was threatening to 'normality', rather than the basis for much-needed rescue. In these narratives, women did not convey an immediate sense that something might 'go wrong', but rather an intuitive belief that if they trusted themselves, their bodies and their caregivers, they would feel safe. Adding weight to Zinn's (2008) argument that individual decisions lie somewhere in between rationality and an emotional or heuristic belief that 'this' is right for them, these accounts still paid homage to the need for a 'safety net', but this was less central, allowing social, emotional and relational factors to be a prime motivation for selecting a particular setting for birth.

Very few women, representing a minority within the smaller group who opted for non-OU birth, actively took issue with the idea that birth was potentially risky and argued a case that birth without medical oversight was safer, suggesting either that the 'natural' birth argument has declined in recent decades, or that the recent proliferation of discourses of risk, blame and responsibility renders such a perspective difficult to voice in contemporary times. This may be out of step with epidemiological evidence that birth is generally very safe (Birthplace in England Collaborative Group 2011), but it remains persistent, and reflects the discourses and uncertainties facing women. These observations raise further questions about whether women are, in practice, able to make decisions that conflict with their immediate cultural reference point, whether this originates in their 'natal' family and nationality or in the cultural public and professional narratives which continue to position birth as risky despite evidence of safety.

Conclusion

Douglas and Wildavsky's (1982) assertion that some risks are politically 'selected' to support a given argument, whilst others are overlooked, is, to some extent, supported in this analysis. However, the term 'risk selection' perhaps suggests too strongly that a conscious decision has been made to focus on particular risks, and to allow this to underpin decision-making. Rather, it would seem that decisions are informed by impressions and understandings gleaned over time, which merge to form a sense of risk, and that individuals may not be immediately aware of the source of their beliefs, feelings and expectations. On the other hand, Douglas and Wildavsky's (1982) observation that the 'line of normality' provides a basis for risk differentiation proves consistently valuable; if hospital OU birth is considered 'normal', then women who elect to birth without doctors present may be held to account if death or mishap occurs. It might then be expected that this view could change if home and other non-OU settings for birth became culturally positioned as 'normal', but given the historical basis of women's beliefs, such a change is unlikely to be rapid or even to occur within a generation. Given the prevailing national and international discourses of birth as predominantly risky, we argue that marginalisation of 'alternative' settings is likely to persist. It also seems likely that expressing views or preferences which are at odds with the prevailing culture will remain difficult, even in high-income countries with good health infrastructure and high-level policy support for birth in settings other than OUs.

Acknowledgements

The views and opinions expressed therein are those of the authors and do not necessarily reflect those of the NIHR, NHS or the Department of Health. We are grateful to those who gave their time and participated in interviews, and to the NHS trusts which supported this research.

Funding

The research was supported by the National Institute of Health Research [NIHR/RTF/08/01/022].

Note

1. The National Childbirth Trust is a UK charity which aims to support parents, through providing information, networking and education for pregnancy and beyond.

References

Abel, S. and Kearns, R.A., 1991. Birth places: a geographical perspective on planned home birth in New Zealand. *Social science and medicine*, 33 (7), 825–834.

Barber, T., Rogers, J.M.S., and Marsh, S., 2006. The birth place choices project: phase one. *British journal of midwifery*, 14 (10), 609–613.

Beck, U., 1992. *Risk society: towards a new modernity*. London: Sage Books.

Birthplace in England Collaborative Group [BPiE], 2011. Perinatal and maternal outcomes by planned place of birth for healthy women with low risk pregnancies: the birthplace in England national prospective cohort study. *British medical journal*, 343, d7400. doi:10.1136/bmj.d7400

Brown, P.R., *et al.*, 2011. Actions speak louder than words: the embodiment of trust by healthcare professionals in gynae-oncology. *Sociology of health and illness*, 33 (2), 280–295.

Bryant, J., *et al.*, 2007. Caesarean birth: consumption, safety, order and good mothering. *Social science and medicine*, 65, 1192–1201.

Bury, M., 2001. Illness narratives: fact or fiction? *Sociology of health and illness*, 23 (3), 263–285.

Cheyney, M.J., 2008. Home birth as systems-challenging praxis: knowledge power and intimacy in the birthplace. *Qualitative health research*, 18 (2), 254–267.

Coxon, K., 2012. *Birth place decisions: a prospective, qualitative study of how women and their partners make sense of risk and safety when choosing where to give birth.* Thesis (PhD). King's College, London.

Cunningham, J.D., 1993. Experiences of Australian mothers who gave birth either at home, at a birth centre, or in hospital labour wards. *Social science and medicine,* 36 (4), 475–483.

Dahlen, H.G. and Homer, C.S.E., 2013. 'Motherbirth or childbirth'? A prospective analysis of vaginal birth after caesarean section blogs. *Midwifery,* 29, 167–173.

Davis-Floyd, R., 1990. The role of obstetric rituals in the resolution of cultural anomaly. *Social science and medicine,* 31 (2), 175–189.

Davis-Floyd, R., 1992. *Birth as an American rite of passage.* Berkeley: University of California Press.

Davis-Floyd, R., 1994. The technocratic body: American childbirth as cultural expression. *Social science and medicine,* 38 (8), 1125–1140.

Davis-Floyd R. and Sargent C., eds., 1997. *Childbirth and authoritative knowledge: cross cultural perspectives.* Berkeley: University of California Press.

Department of Health [DH], 1993. *Changing childbirth: report of the expert maternity group.* London: HMSO.

Department of Health [DH], 2007. *Maternity matters: choice, access and continuity of care in a safe service.* London: The Stationery Office.

DeVries, R., *et al.,* 2001. What (and why) do women want? The desires of women and the design of maternity care. *In*: R. DeVries, *et al.,* eds. *Birth by design: pregnancy, maternity care and midwifery in North America and Europe.* London: Routledge. 243–266.

Donner, H., 2003. The place of birth: childbearing and kinship in Calcutta middle-class families. *Medical anthropology,* 22, 303–341.

Douglas, M., 1966/2002. *Purity and danger.* Oxon: Routledge Classics Edition Routledge. [First published 1966].

Douglas, M., 1970/2003. *Natural symbols.* 2nd ed. Oxon: Routledge Classics Edition, Routledge. [First published 1970].

Douglas, M. and Wildavsky, A., 1982. *Risk and culture: an essay on the selection of technical and environmental dangers.* Berkeley: University of California Press.

Edwards, N., 2005. *Birthing autonomy: women's experience of home births.* London: Routledge.

Ehrich, K., 2003. Reconceptualizing 'inappropriateness': researching multiple moral positions in demand for primary healthcare. *Health,* 7 (1), 109–126.

Fahy, K., Foureur, M., and Hastie, C., eds., 2008. *Birth territory and midwifery guardianship: theory for practice, education and research.* Edinburgh: Butterworth Heinemann Elsevier.

Garcia, J., Kilpatrick, R., and Richards, M., eds., 1990. *The politics of maternity care: services for childbearing women in twentieth-century Britain.* Oxford: Clarendon Press.

Giddens, A., 1991. *Modernity and self-identify: self and society in the late modern age.* Cambridge: Polity Press.

Green, J., 1999. From accidents to risk: public health and preventable injury. *Health, risk & society,* 1 (1), 25–39. doi:10.1080/13698579908407005

Health Care Commission [HCC], 2008. *Towards better births: a review of maternity services in England.* London: Commission for Healthcare Audit and Inspection.

Henwood, K.L., *et al.,* 2010. Researching risk: narrative, biography, subjectivity. *Forum: qualitative social research,* 11 (1). Art. 20. Available from: http://www.qualitative-research. net/index.php/fqs/article/view/1438/2926 [Accessed 11 November 2013].

Hodnett, E.D., *et al.,* 2010. Alternative versus conventional institutional settings for birth. *Cochrane database of systematic reviews,* Issue 9. Art. No.: CD000012. doi: 10.1002/14651858. CD000012.pub3 (Citation as instructed).

Houghton, G., *et al.,* 2008. Factors influencing choice in birth place – an exploration of the views of women, their partners and professionals. *Evidence based midwifery,* 6 (2), 59–64.

Inch, S., 1982. *Birthrights.* London: Hutchinson.

Kitzinger, S., 2005. *The politics of birth.* Oxford: Butterworth Heinemann.

Lancet, 1963. Perinatal mortality. *Lancet,* 282 (7319), 1207–1208.

Lee, E.J., 2008. Living with risk in the age of 'intensive motherhood': maternal identity and infant feeding. *Health, risk & society,* 10 (5), 467–477.

Lee, S., Ayers, S., and Holden, D., 2012. Risk perception of women during high risk pregnancy: a systematic review. *Health, risk & society,* 14 (6), 511–531.

Liamputtong, P., 2005. Birth and social class: northern Thai women's lived experiences of caesarean and vaginal birth. *Sociology of health and illness*, 27 (2), 243–270.

Mansfield, B., 2008. The social nature of natural childbirth. *Social science and medicine*, 66, 1084–1094.

Marshall, H. and Woollett, A., 2000. Fit to reproduce? The regulatory role of pregnancy texts. *Feminism & psychology*, 10 (3), 351–366.

Miller, T., 2011. *Making sense of fatherhood: gender, caring and work*. Cambridge: Cambridge University Press.

Murray, S.F. and Elston, M.A., 2005. The promotion of private health insurance and its implications for the social organisation of healthcare: a case study of private sector obstetric practice in Chile. *Sociology of health and illness*, 27 (6), 701–721.

Nash, M., 2011. 'You don't train for a marathon sitting on a couch': performances of pregnancy 'fitness' and 'good' motherhood in Melbourne, Australia. *Women's studies international forum*, 34, 50–65.

National Collaborating Centre for Women's and Children's Health [NCCWCH], 2007. *Intrapartum care: care of healthy women and their babies during childbirth*. Clinical Guideline 55. London: RCOG Press. Available from: http://publications.nice.org.uk/intrapartum-care-cg55/guidance#planning-place-of-birth [Accessed 26 July 2012].

Nelson, M., 1983. Working-class women, middle-class women and models of childbirth. *Social problems*, 30 (3), 284–297.

Office for National Statistics [ONS], 2009. *Statistical bulletin: who is having babies? (2008)*. London: ONS.

Patton, M.Q., 2002. *Qualitative research & evaluation methods*. 3rd ed. Thousands Oaks, CA: Sage.

Pitchforth, E., *et al.*, 2008. Models of intrapartum care and women's trade-offs in remote and rural Scotland: a mixed methods study. *British journal of obstetrics and gynaecology*, 115, 560–569.

Pitchforth, E., *et al.*, 2009. 'Choice' and place of delivery; a qualitative study of women in remote and rural Scotland. *Quality and safety in health care*, 18, 42–48.

Redshaw, M., *et al.*, 2011. Mapping maternity care: the configuration of maternity care in England. Birthplace in England research programme. Final report part 3. NIHR Service Delivery and Organisation programme.

Riessman, C.K., 2008. *Narrative methods for the human sciences*. Thousand Oaks, CA: Sage.

Rowe, R., 2011. *Birthplace terms and definitions: consensus process*. Birthplace in England Research Programme. London: NIHR Service Delivery and Organisation Programme, Final Report Part 2.

Royal College of Obstetricians and Gynaecologists [RCOG], 2013. *Patterns of variation in maternity care in English NHS hospitals*. London: Royal College of Obstetricians and Gynaecologists.

Scamell, M., 2011. The swan effect in midwifery talk and practice: a tension between normality and the language of risk. *Sociology of health and illness*, 33 (7), 987–1001.

Scamell, M. and Alaszewski, A., 2012. Fateful moments and the categorisation of risk: midwifery practice and the ever-narrowing window of normality during birth. *Health, risk & society*, 14 (20), 207–221.

Taylor-Gooby, P.F., ed., 2000. *Risk trust and welfare*. Basingstoke: Palgrave Macmillan.

Topliss, E., 1970. Selection procedure for hospital and domiciliary confinements. *In*: G. McLachlan and R. Shegog, eds. *In the beginning: studies of maternity services*. London: Oxford University Press, 59–78.

Viisainen, K., 2000. The moral dangers of home birth: parents' perceptions of risks in home birth in Finland. *Sociology of health and illness*, 22 (6), 792–814.

Viisainen, K., 2001. Negotiating control and meaning: home birth as a self-constructed choice in Finland. *Social science and medicine*, 52 (7), 1109–1121.

Wengraf, T., 2001. *Qualitative research interviewing: biographic narrative and semi-structured method*. London: Sage.

Zadoroznyj, M., 1999. Social class, social selves and social control in childbirth. *Sociology of health and illness*, 21 (3), 267–289.

Zinn, J.O., 2008. Heading into the unknown: everyday strategies for managing risk and uncertainty. *Health, risk & society*, 10 (5), 439–450. doi:10.1080/13698570802380891

Negotiating risky bodies: childbirth and constructions of risk

Rachelle Joy Chadwick[a] and Don Foster[b]

[a]Women's Health Research Unit, University of Cape Town, Cape Town, South Africa; [b]Department of Psychology, University of Cape Town, Cape Town, South Africa

Policy makers, practitioners and researchers have identified risk as a key concept in relation to maternity care and childbirth. There is however a lack of research exploring women's discursive constructions of risk and childbirth in relation to sociological risk theories. In this article we explore pregnant women's everyday negotiations of risk in relation to the self-chosen plan to birth either at home or via an elective Caesarean section. We use sociocultural risk theories to contextualise our findings. This article draws on data from a study conducted in 2005–2006 in which we interviewed 24 pregnant middle-class South African women who were planning a home birth or elective Caesarean section and used social constructionist discourse analysis to analyse the data. We found that women's risk constructions were related to three different conceptions of birthing embodiment: technocratic bodies, vulnerable bodies and knowing bodies. Women who planned Caesarean sections were committed to biomedical constructions of risk and birth. Woman who planned home births shifted between endorsing and subverting biomedical models of risk. They also resisted definitions of birthing bodies as inherently abject (unclean, polluting, unruly) and constructed the process of giving birth as risky in medicalised settings. In such settings, the birthing body was constructed as vulnerable to objectification, loss of dignity and shaming. Women who planned to give birth at home constructed an alternative approach to birth which emphasised embodied ways of knowing, relational connection and empowerment over normative and medicalised risk constructions. In the process, biomedical risk definitions were destabilised.

Introduction

In this article, we examine the ways in which 24 pregnant middle-class South African women negotiated and constructed risk in the context of talking about their plan to give birth either at home or via an elective Caesarean section. There are extensive debates in the literature regarding the concept of childbirth 'choices' in relation to elective Caesarean section and home birth (see for example Kingdon et al. 2003, McCourt et al. 2004, Edwards 2005, Boucher et al. 2009, Munro et al. 2009, Fenwick et al. 2010, Karlström et al. 2011), and we have published on this aspect of our data elsewhere (see Chadwick and Foster 2013). In this article we focus on risk constructions and aim to add to the literature on the 'lived experience' of risk (Lupton 1999a) by investigating the ways in which pregnant middle-class South African women positioned themselves in relation to the possible risks of childbirth.

Risk and childbirth

Approaches to risk

Risk theorists argue that we live in a 'risk society' (Beck 1992) defined by increasing and pervasive risks. These risks are the product of modern society and dominant institutions such as industry, science and government, but the responsibility for risk management has become individualised. As individuals we have access to a wide array of knowledge and the freedom to make choices and negotiate risks. As a result, 'risk consciousness' (Lupton 2012) has become an integral part of individual subjectivities.

The field of 'risk theory' is rich and complex. Lupton (1999b) however provides a broad and flexible approach to diverse theoretical positions on risk. In this overview (see Lupton 1999a, 1999b), she argues that the 'technico-scientific' approach is the hegemonic model of risk, conceptualising risks as objective phenomena which can be predicted and controlled via science and expert knowledge. In contrast to this there are various 'sociocultural' theories of risk, including Beck's 'risk society' theory, the cultural-symbolic approach of Mary Douglas and Foucauldian governmentality (Lupton 1999b). Sociocultural approaches conceptualise hazards as shaped by social and cultural norms and as historically and locally variable (Lupton and Tulloch 2002a). While the subject conceptualised by a 'risk society' approach is a rational, autonomous agent/consumer who has the freedom to choose their responses to risk knowledges, the Foucauldian subject is infiltrated by power and moral technologies of risk and becomes a 'self-regulating moral agent' who actively participates in regimes of regulation as part of the project of selfhood (Lupton 1999a, p. 104). The cultural-symbolic approach of Douglas is less concerned with individuals and more interested in risk as a strategy for policing symbolic boundaries between self/other and different social groups. Risk is thus politicised (Lupton 1999b) and seen as a means of maintaining social order and cohesion (Tulloch and Lupton 2003). These three sociocultural approaches to risk tend to operate at the level of 'grand theory' with little effort to explore everyday risk constructions (Lupton 1999b).

As a result, Lupton (1999a) identifies phenomenological/hermeneutic approaches to risk as empirical work interested in exploring the 'lived experience' of risk or situated and local meaning-making. In addition to providing a broad overview of risk theories, Lupton and colleagues have conducted a range of studies investigating the micro-analytics of risk, the socially constructed nature of risk epistemologies (ways of knowing about risk) and counter discourses of risk (Lupton and Tulloch 1998, Lupton and Tulloch 2002a, 2002b, Lupton 2011). Associated with qualitative methodologies, this body of risk research is interested in the micro-context of risk and its relationship to normative discourses and power relations. Thus, while sociocultural risk theory largely assumes risk to be negative with risk-avoidant behaviours regarded as normal, micro-analytic work has shown that the situated meanings of risk are complex and that risk can be associated with pleasure and positiveness for individuals (Lupton and Tulloch 2002a, 2002b, Tulloch and Lupton 2003). Furthermore, micro-analytic work on risk has also shown the complexities of lay risk knowledges as 'situated rationalities' (Tulloch and Lupton 2003, p. 9) which compete with expert knowledges. For example, experiential forms of knowledge such as intuition are regarded by many people as the most trustworthy source of information in relation to risk (Tulloch and Lupton 2003).

Risk in childbirth

Nowhere is the pervasiveness of risk more apparent than in the sphere of pregnancy and childbirth (Smith *et al.* 2012). With technological advances in reproductive medicine, the concept of risk has increasingly over the last 40 years come to define women's experiences of pregnancy and childbirth (Helén 2004). While childbirth has become safer than ever for women in developed world contexts, risk discourses have paradoxically intensified (Lankshear *et al.* 2005, Possamai-Inesedy 2006). In most countries childbirth has been redefined as a medical event with obstetric science promising to predict and minimise its risks. While a large corpus of feminist literature has critiqued the biomedical model of childbirth and argued that it disempowers birthing women and renders a normal event pathological (Rothman 1982, Martin 1987, Davis-Floyd and Sargent 1997), studies have shown that many women embrace biomedical forms of birth (Fox and Worts 1999; Davis-Floyd 2003). Technocratic models of childbirth knowledge are authoritative (Jordan 1997) and hegemonic, increasingly even in developing world contexts (Davis-Floyd 2003).

The language of risk permeates biomedical models of childbirth which operate largely within a 'technico-scientific' model of risk emphasising expert and evidence-based knowledge, prediction and control (Lupton 1999b). To minimise risk, childbirth must therefore be managed by experts, constantly monitored and is subject to a series of investigations in order to probe dysfunction and abnormality. While the dominance of risk discourse in relation to childbirth is widely accepted (Hausman 2005, Mackenzie Bryers and van Teijlingen 2010, Smith *et al.* 2012), few studies have utilised risk theory to explore everyday constructions of risk and childbirth. This is surprising given that several studies have explored the intersections between pregnancy and risk (Lupton 1999c, 2012, Ruhl 1999, Root and Browner 2001, McDonald *et al.* 2011) infant feeding and risk (Law 2000, Murphy 2004, Lee 2007a, 2007b, 2008, Knaak 2010) and parenting and risk (Murphy 2003, Lupton 2008, 2011, Kelhä 2009) within the rubric of sociological risk theories.

While a key issue in studies of childbirth, 'risk' is rarely critically examined; it is equated with medically defined risks, and the possibility of iatrogenic risks arising from the use of medical procedures is largely ignored (see Hausman 2005, Seibold *et al.* 2010). There have been studies that have investigated the construction of risk in midwifery practice, utilising ethnographic methods to explore the everyday work and discourse of midwives (e.g. Annandale 1988, Lankshear *et al.* 2005, Seibold *et al.* 2010, Scamell 2011, Scamell and Alaszewski 2012). These studies have found that despite a commitment to normal birth, midwives remain preoccupied with discourses of biomedical risk, surveillance and the dangers of childbirth. According to Scamell and Alaszewski (2012), normality in childbirth is increasingly an absent signifier and has 'no language of its own' (p. 216) in the discourse of midwives.

There is a lack of research exploring the construction of risk in women's own discourse about childbirth, though there are exceptions. For example, Possamai-Inesedy (2006) found that a discourse of biomedical risk suffused Australian women's talk about childbirth. Her study included a sample of women who gave birth in different locations (private hospital, birth centre, home birth), but she found that biomedical risk discourses dominated with little evidence of alternative constructions. Other studies have however found women's constructions of risk and childbirth to be more complex. For example, Miller and Shriver (2012) found that American women's definitions of risk differed according to their 'birth habitus'. 'Habitus' refers to the term drawn from the sociological theory of Pierre Bourdieu (2005, p. 43) and refers to a 'system of dispositions' in which particular social contexts, such as class, produce ways of being, perceiving and acting in the world. Women located within a 'scientific-medical habitus' defined risk in conventional biomedical terms, while women located in other modes of habitus (for example a religious or natural family habitus) defined safety and risk in non-medical terms. Lindgren *et al.* (2008) drew on data from a questionnaire survey that examined the risk perceptions of 735 Swedish women who gave birth at home. They found that women associated hospital birth with risks involving loss of autonomy, being amongst strangers, subject to possible unnecessary interventions and a foreign hospital environment. Edwards and Murphy-Lawless (2006) conducted an interview study of 30 Scottish women who gave birth at home and found that biomedical definitions of risk were challenged, with many aspects of medicalised birth constructed as risky, such as invasive procedures, loss of autonomy and being forced to comply with generalised obstetric norms and timetables. Viisainen's (2000) qualitative study of 21 Finnish women who gave birth at home found that women identified biomedical, iatrogenic and moral issues in their talk about risk. Moral concerns related to the possibility of stigma and social censure in a Finnish context in which hospital birth was equated with safety and home birth with danger. However, women balanced these concerns by emphasising the possible iatrogenic harm from medical interventions and presented this as their main justification for a home birth.

Choice of birth and risk in South Africa

Medicalised birth is the dominant mode of childbirth in South Africa, with 93.5% of women giving birth in a hospital or obstetric unit (South African Demographic and Health Survey 2003, 2007). Self-chosen home birth and elective Caesarean section are atypical birth choices in the South African context. Childbirth is divided along racial lines, with 51% of white women giving birth with specialist gynaecologists or obstetricians in highly resourced private hospitals and approximately 84% of black women giving birth with midwives in poorly resourced public hospitals or midwife-obstetric units (South African Demographic and Health Survey 2003, 2007). In South Africa, there is little research and no available national figures on planned home birth. Clear figures reporting the incidence of elective Caesarean section for personal reasons are unavailable in the South African context. Small studies however indicate that between 8.7% (Naidoo and Moodley 2009) and 35.6% (Lawrie *et al.* 2001) of Caesareans are elective. It is not clear what proportion of these are medically necessary procedures or due to maternal request.

Currently there is little research on risk in South Africa, so in our study and analysis, we have drawn on Lupton's (1999a, 1999b) overview of sociocultural risk theories. While there are no known investigations of risk and birth in South Africa, there is evidence that biomedical 'technico-scientific' models of risk are becoming hegemonic in other developing world contexts such as Mexico, Brazil, Ghana and China (see Diniz and Chacham 2004, Bogg *et al.* 2010, Denham 2012, Smith-Oka 2012). Middle-class birthing in South Africa, the context for our study, is highly medicalised and marked by one of the highest Caesarean section rates in the world. Caesarean section rates in private hospitals are estimated to range between 40% and 82% (Tshibangu *et al.* 2002, Rothberg and Macleod 2005, Naidoo and Moodley 2009).

In this article we focus on everyday risk constructions in relation to the choice to birth at home or via an elective Caesarean section. We aim to add to the literature on the 'lived experience' of risk (Lupton 1999a) by investigating the ways in which pregnant middle-class South African women construct risk in relation to childbirth choices. It is important to focus on women's perspectives on risk and childbirth in order to explore the ways in which normative biomedical definitions of risk are potentially reproduced or challenged in everyday discursive practice.

Method

In this article we draw on interview data from a feminist discursive research project interested in childbirth agency and birth narratives in the context of planned home birth and Caesarean section. We examine how women discursively constructed risk and positioned themselves in relation to normative definitions of biomedical risk.

Design and approach

Since we wanted to explore how women constructed risk in relation to birth, we used a social constructionist form of discourse analysis to examine the constructive features of women's talk about childbirth and risk (see Parker 1992). Discourse analysis is a 'theory-method' (Potter 1997) concerned with the material and ideological power of language to construct realities, 'truths' and subjectivities. Social constructionist discourse analysis treats talk and text as primary analytic objects and is thus not concerned with the underlying motivations or intentions of individual agents. Parker (1992, pp. 8–9) describes discourses as 'sets of meanings which constitute objects' and which offer spaces for 'particular types of selves' to materialise. Parker's (1992) discourse analytic framework, located within a Foucauldian tradition of discourse analysis, was used to identify key risk discourses and interrogate the kinds of realities and subjectivities these discourses produced. We followed Parker's (1992) analytic steps which included identifying the objects (for example natural birth, Caesarean section, female bodies, risk) and subjects (such as birthing women, doctors, midwives) in the transcript texts. Questions were asked about how these objects and subjects were constituted, as well as what rights to speak or 'voice' was accorded to subjects identified in the transcript texts. We looked for points of contradiction in order to facilitate the identification of different discourses or 'sets of meanings' about risk, birth and women's bodies (Parker 1992, pp. 8–9).

Pre- and post-birth interviews were conducted with 24 women in 2005–2006. Pre-birth interviews were semi-structured and focussed on women's experience of pregnancy, their rationale for their respective birth choice and expectations about the upcoming birth. Post-birth interviews focused on women's birth narratives and were largely unstructured in order to encourage storytelling. These interviews began with the broad question, 'what happened with the birth?' and proceeded largely as informal conversations. Almost all of the interviews took place in participant's homes. One participant preferred to be interviewed in the workplace. Interviews lasted between 45 minutes and 2 hours. The interviews were conducted, transcribed and analysed by the first author (Rachelle Chadwick). In this article we draw mainly on the pre-birth interviews which were conducted when women were approximately 7 months pregnant. We make more limited use of the data from the post-birth interviews which occurred at approximately 6 weeks after the birth.

Our analysis involved careful repeated readings of interview transcripts to identify dominant and transgressive discourses of risk. The key issues we addressed in the texts were:

- How was risk constructed in women's talk?
- What forms of knowledge underpinned risk constructions?
- How were women constituted as subjects in talk about risk?
- How was embodiment reproduced and negotiated in risk discourse?
- Were there subversive and contradictory discourses in relation to risk constructions present in women's talk?

Sampling and data collection

We decided to focus on middle-class women who could afford private maternity care and were planning on atypical modes of birth in the South African context. We were able to recruit 24 middle-class women who had chosen either to give birth at home (*n* = 15) or have an elective Caesarean section (*n* = 9). We had to use a snowball method to recruit participants given the difficulty of locating pregnant women who were planning to give birth at home or via maternal request Caesarean section. Letters were placed in local community newspapers and a national pregnancy magazine inviting potential participants to take part in the study. The first author (Rachelle Chadwick) also contacted local private midwives and asked for help in locating pregnant women planning home births. She gave talks at antenatal classes at four private hospitals inviting women who were planning to have a Caesarean for personal reasons to take part in the research. Most of the women (11 out of 15) who had chosen to give birth at home were recruited through private midwives (*n* = 11), while most women (5 out of 9) planning an elective Caesarean were recruited via visits to antenatal classes. All but one of the women planning home births gave birth at home, and all of the women planning Caesareans gave birth via elective Caesarean section. One woman changed her mind about her planned home birth and decided to give birth in a birth centre instead.

The women who volunteered to take part were predominantly white (22 out of 24), with two women of mixed racial descent. The average age of participants was 33 years, and all of the women (except one woman choosing to give birth at home) were involved in long-term relationships. One woman indicated that her pregnancy was unplanned. Most of the women choosing to give birth at home were expecting their second or third baby (13 out of 15), while all but one of the nine women choosing Caesarean sections were expecting their first baby. All of the women gave birth without complications. We obtained ethical approval for the study from the Department of Psychology at the University of Cape Town and used standard ethical principles of informed consent, anonymity and confidentiality. All the names used in this article are pseudonyms.

Findings

In this section we draw on our discursive analysis of women's talk about their birth choices (elective Caesarean or home birth) to examine the ways in which risk was constructed in relation to birth.

Technocratic bodies and biomedical forms of knowing

Women choosing elective Caesareans positioned themselves within biomedical forms of knowing about childbirth. Choosing a Caesarean section was itself constructed as a form of risk management. In line with a technico-scientific model of risk, obstetric risks in the form of complications and abnormalities were cast as manageable with expert knowledge and maximum degrees of technological monitoring and intervention. All of these women used specialist gynaecologists or obstetricians and had an ultrasound with each visit to their doctor. Some of the women went for extra monitoring at a local 'foetal assessment centre', and two had amniocentesis testing. They regarded the use of midwives as caregivers during pregnancy/childbirth as inherently dangerous because of their associated low levels of technocratic monitoring. For example, Lola drew on her personal knowledge of a friend in England who had not had the benefits of access to the full range of medical technology which she had in South Africa:

Lola: I'm fairly scared of midwives. (laughing) I must tell you, I had a friend over there [in England] that had a baby and they scan I think, through the whole pregnancy, they did three scans, so the pregnancy is not monitored as well as is done over here and um there were complications and the baby was, the baby wasn't normal and they only picked that up late in the pregnancy, which I think over here would have been picked up quite soon, so things like that I think is more or less ruled out over here.

In this extract, technocratic monitoring is constructed as a means of identifying and controlling potential 'risks' in the form of foetal abnormalities. However, it remains unclear whether it is 'abnormal' babies or belated diagnoses that are eliminated by regular monitoring. The implication is however that technoscience can predict and thus help to control risks of abnormality, deformity and disease.

The women who decided to have an elective Caesarean constructed it as 'a safer choice' than vaginal delivery. In their discourse, childbirth was constructed as inherently risky and dangerous. As a result, an elective Caesarean and a highly technocratic approach was seen as the 'safest' way to deal with uncertainties and guarantee a positive outcome. For women choosing Caesareans, risks and dangers came from the 'natural' birth process and the female reproductive body itself. Technology was seen as the solution to risk and never as a potential complicating factor. These women used a language of biomedical risk to talk about their birth choices, with medical technology seen as the key means of managing risks. For Hannalie, technology was a way of managing 'too many things that can go wrong':

Hannalie: She [sister-in-law] had a normal birth the first time and then the second time the baby was overdue two weeks, and only the morning when they did the induction and they put the heart monitor on, did they realise that this baby has been in distress because there's no amniotic fluid left and then they realised if they don't take the baby out now, it's not going to survive, and then I ask myself now what would have happened if they didn't, you know, if they didn't put the monitor on? You know, so I dunno, I think these things should be controlled, it's, it's, there's just too many things that can go wrong.

For Janine as for Hannalie, a Caesarean section was seen as the best way of managing the uncertainty of childbirth:

Janine: You dunno know how long it's [natural birth] gonna last, you dunno if you're going to end up having a Caesar in any case so ja, you just don't know what, what's going to happen.

Hannalie: Lying there for 8 to 12 hours, not knowing what's going on, would drive me insane, there's too much uncertainty, there's too many variables.

These extracts show an investment in technocratic forms of knowledge in which prediction and control are prioritised over the uncertainties created by extraneous 'variables'. For women choosing Caesareans, surgical birth was construed as the ultimate expression of technico-scientific knowledge and its ability to conquer risk and unpredictability. According to Karin, a Caesarean section 'really fitted into my paradigm of knowing'. Furthermore, the 'end-product' of birth, namely the baby, was regarded as more important than the process of birth, which was seen as just a means to an end. For women choosing Caesareans, the process or experience of childbirth had little intrinsic worth or value. Thus, according to Hannalie, 'What's the point of natural birth?'

For women who chose to have a Caesarean section the procedure itself was seen as evidence of technico-scientific progress. Caesarean sections was cast as a modern, civilised and technologically advanced form of childbirth. For example, Caroline linked Caesarean sections to the progress of modern medicine:

Caroline: You know I think we've progressed with modern medicine and it's [a Caesarean] for me, a choice that makes sense to me, you know, we've progressed.

Similarly, for Hannalie, 'normal birth' was old-fashioned and out of date, while Caesarean sections were modern and part of medical advances:

Hannalie: I mean, medical procedures have advanced so much today, if you look at the way they do a heart operation, they do it differently to the way they did it ten years ago. Why would you then go the normal route, if you, why would you go the old route of a heart operation, if you can go the new route? Why would you have a normal birth if you can have a Caesarean section?

Women choosing Caesareans were thus deeply committed to a positivist paradigm of science and technology as the path to conquering obstetric risk and complications.

Regardless of their birth choice, all the women in our study constructed biomedically defined risks as salient in relation to childbirth. Many of the women who had chosen to give birth at home talked about the riskiness of their decision. For example, Stephanie, who would be defined as 'high-risk' according to conventional obstetrics because of her age, described the difficulties of making the decision to have her first baby at home and the reassurance which medical technology afforded her during her second pregnancy:

Stephanie: Um, it [decision to have first birth at home] was very challenged by, then I was 37 and first birth, just literally um culturally that negativity that, that um challenged my confidence quite often, I would feel, 'Am I doing the right thing?' 'What if something goes wrong?' You know, how can I homebirth and then something goes wrong? .... This time round we had huge angst about twins, we went for scans, you need to know, I mean it's a huge economic thing, um, and being gradually worn down by nausea and feeling 'Am I going to do this?' and 'I'm 42 years old and what if this is a Downs Syndrome baby?' 'What if? What if? What if?' I went for an 18 week scan which was fascinating, once I gave over to it you know, this has a place and it has meaning, um, to know whether there was abnormality.

Women who planned to give birth at home thus strategically drew on medical technology to identify and manage fears and uncertainties. Most (similarly to women in Kornelsen's (2005) study) were not opposed to technology per se but rather to unnecessary interventions. However, some women were more opposed to technology than others. For example, Angela was against all forms of technology, including ultrasounds and argued that the possible dangers of such procedures were not fully known:

Angela: I think the more one interferes the more likely that there is damage in the baby, you know they say it's [ultrasound] linked to remedial difficulties and they don't actually know, I mean scanning hasn't been around that long, they don't know the side-effects.

In this extract, Angela overturns technocratic risk discourse and constructs medical experts as not having full knowledge and technology itself as potentially risky and dangerous. Other women who chose to give birth at home also questioned the validity of the knowledge created by medical technology. For example, Jane refused to have an ultrasound after her (only) scan at 22 weeks because she did not trust the results and felt they created unnecessary problems:

> Jane: I don't have scans at 36 weeks because then they start telling you 'Oh your baby's so big and your baby's this and your baby's that' and I'm like – 'No, thank you'.

In contrast to women choosing Caesareans, most women who had home births engaged in the minimum of technocratic 'monitoring' such as ultrasounds, with none having more invasive testing such as amniocentesis. Some, like Anke, however, wanted to have 'the best of both worlds'. She consulted a gynaecologist, a midwife and a 'sonar specialist' specialising in 3D ultrasounds to make sure that all was well and she could go ahead with her plan to give birth at home.

In the talk of women choosing Caesareans, biomedical risk discourse was used as a rationale for their birth choice. In their discourse, 'natural' childbirth was constructed as risky and dangerous, while the potential risks of Caesarean sections were minimised. Instead, the safety, predictability and controllable aspects of Caesarean sections were emphasised by women. Caroline did however acknowledge the risks of having a Caesarean but felt that these were minimal in the South African context:

> Caroline: I think um medically, if you haven't got a good surgeon or, anything can go wrong your, your spinal block, any of those things, there, there are certainly big risks involved but I, I just, I think medically I think we've got I think, I think the risks are less, just where we are, maybe if I was in a different country, I, if I was up in Africa and someone wanted to do a Caesar, I don't know if I'd want to do that (laughs) I think I'd, I might just go the natural route or something ... but I think where we live and our medical expertise, I think there's less, there's less risk in a Caesar nowadays.

Caroline thus concedes that Caesareans are risky – 'anything can go wrong'. However, she also constructs the procedure as 'less risky' in the context of the highly specialised medical expertise available in the private maternity sector in South Africa (to affluent patients).

Vulnerable bodies and the risks of (medicalised) birth

While obstetric risk in the form of abnormalities, complications and possible death (particularly of the infant) was ever-present in women's discourse, there was another category of risk evident in their talk about making birth choices. This risk centred around the status/treatment of the birthing body itself. For women negotiating childbirth choices, the potential status/treatment of the birthing body featured as a major source of risk.

Childbirth is an event in which bodily boundaries potentially break down and in which the 'proper', civilised and individualised body threatens to become open, volatile and multiple. Childbirth is thus a potentially threatening form of embodiment that is, as a result, subject to social control and policing (Lupton 1999a). In technocratic societies, social control over birth occurs largely though medicalised childbirth rituals (see Davis-Floyd 2003). The women in this study recognised the inherent threats and vulnerabilities of birthing embodiment, including loss of bodily control and mistreatment. For women choosing Caesareans, threats of loss of bodily control, leaking bodies (blood, sweat, urine, faeces, amniotic fluid), fragmenting bodies (tearing, stretching) and fears about being reduced to a form of primitive animality during labour/delivery emerged as a key risk in relation to childbirth. For example, Karin noted that she did not want to lose bodily control in front of other people:

> Karin: I don't want the risks associated with tearing, I don't want to push and sweat and moan and swear, I don't want to lie and pooh [defecate] in front of anyone.

Hannalie equated 'normal' birth with degrading animal-like behaviour which would be witnessed by strangers:

> Hannalie: My one friend said to me, 'it's um, it's an embarrassing process to go through, to give normal birth, because you've got no control, you, you're left to these people [medical staff] and you have to lie in an obscene position and it's animal-like'.

For these women, childbirth was a threat to bodily integrity, an 'uncontrollable materiality' (Grosz 1989, p. 72) that induced a kind of abject horror and disgust. For women who have internalised the values of technocratic society and the ideal of the autonomous, self-regulated, controlled and 'civilised' body-self, the bodily state of birthing poses a serious threat (Lupton 1999c). The very idea of having to trust in one's body to give birth was difficult for some women to imagine. For example, Hannalie saw 'normal birth' as a nightmare:

> Hannalie: I think it will be a nightmarish experience for me, if I have to go into labour and have to now rely on my body to produce this baby (laughing) uggghh, no.

All the women in our study were concerned about the vulnerabilities of the birthing body and the preservation of their privacy and dignity during childbirth. While women who chose Caesareans saw the embodied experience of birth as itself threatening, undignified, obscene and horrifying, women who planned home births saw this as a danger of hospital birth that could be avoided through a home birth. Dangers linked to hospitalised birth included being vulnerable to unnecessary interventions and a loss of control and dignity. For example, Lizette equated home birth with being dignified and empowered while hospital birth was filled with uncertainties:

> Lizette: The home birth is so that I can make sure that nobody's going to take him away, that it will be gentle, it will be quiet, um, that I can move around and do what I need to do ... so ja [yes] it's to try and stay out of that whole scenario [hospital birth] and when you go through those doors, of a hospital, your chances are, if you go through those doors you have a 65 per cent chance of having a c-section, 65 per cent chance.

For Jane, being in hospital would mean that male doctors would look at intimate and private parts of her body:

> Jane: Um, I didn't want to be at the mercy of a million doctors lying on my back with my legs up in the air, it's like 'no way', not going there, um ja [yes], and also I don't like the idea of a male doctor looking at my bits you know (laughs).

For women who chose to give birth at home, hospitalised birth was associated with the risks of loss of dignity, objectification and loss of control over decision-making. All the women in our study wanted to protect their bodily vulnerability during birth and retain bodily integrity, dignity and the right to bodily privacy. Women who chose to have home births wanted to avoid the objectifying and potentially undignified treatment of the birthing body in a technocratic, hospital context. For women choosing Caesareans, surgical birth was a way of escaping the uncontrollable, vulnerable and threatening embodiment of birth and retaining control as a rational, disembodied self.

Knowing bodies and childbirth

While women who chose Caesareans unequivocally accepted biomedical definitions of childbirth and its risks, women who chose to have home births veered between acceptance and resistance. One way in which they resisted was by constructing the birthing body as a knowing body rather than the object of medical technology or the site of 'uncontrollable materiality' (Grosz 1989, p. 72). Their articulation of this alternative co-existed with their commitment to biomedical risk discourse. There was thus no pure form of resistance to biomedical definitions of risk. Giving birth at home brought medicalised technologies and surveillance (internal examinations, blood pressure checks, entonox gas for pain relief, injection, resuscitation and suturing equipment) right into women's homes. Furthermore, women who gave birth at home were attuned to issues of obstetric risk and always qualified their choice to have a home birth in relation to medical risk and safety. For example, even Angela, the most vehement 'anti-technology' participant in the study, made regular disclaimers in her interview indicating her ultimate acceptance of technocratic norms, such as: 'but one needs to have some form of back-up' and 'look if I need to go to the hospital, I will ... I'm not going to be stupid about it'.

However, in the midst of these contradictions, women who gave birth at home were engaged in constructing an alternative approach to birth. Similar to what others have termed a 'midwifery model' (see for example Rothman 1982, Klassen 2001), this alternative emerged as a fluid approach consistently placing the birthing woman at the centre of the birth process. This contrasts sharply with a technocratic model of childbirth in which the birthing woman, and her body, feature predominantly as objects of expert knowledge and the passive recipients of technologies to reduce risk. This alternative was grounded in connectedness over risk and privileged forms of knowing produced in/through the birthing body and in connection with others. Women who gave birth at home thus made reference to 'bodily knowing', intuition, 'nature', instinct and the spiritual realm as sources of alternative knowledge. Knowing was often portrayed as an on-going and fluid journey or process. For example, Stephanie described coming to home birth as a journey involving a rediscovery of forms of knowing that had, in her words, 'gone to sleep':

Stephanie: It opened a whole exploration which is where 'Immaculate deception' and a few other things that I got hold of to read and a midwife like Serena were, were essential because it was a whole, in a way an education, but a re-evoking the natural way that I didn't know, that I intuitively knew, um, so a lot of that kind of reading and really just listening to an inner wisdom, and inner knowing, that there is another way, I had a natural capacity to do this thing.

In this extract, Stephanie constructs an alternative model of birth which emphasises the capacities of women as birth givers rather than the source of potential risks/dangers. Knowledge is situated centrally inside the pregnant/birthing body and is realised through connection with others. The birthing body emerges in this extract as a knowing and capable body in contrast to the risky body constructed by technocratic models of birth.

Women who had experienced previous hospital births made it clear that the birthing body emerged as a different entity in the home birth context. For example, Maggie described the ways in which her body was empowered during home birth:

> Maggie: In hospital you know it was, you're lying in stirrups, it's, like it's pure anticipation, so like 'When's the baby going to come out?' and it actually seems to take a lot longer whereas at home it's, your body tells you exactly where it needs to be.

While biomedical discourse defines the birthing body as a site of unpredictability, loss of control and risk, women who birthed at home provided an alternative construction of the birthing body as a site of knowledge and an active capacity. The articulation of birthing bodies as 'knowing bodies' destabilises biomedical conceptualisations of the birthing body as solely a source of risk and potential dysfunction.

Discussion

In this article we have explored middle-class South African women's constructions of risk in relation to the choice to birth at home or via an elective Caesarean section. We found that a 'technico-scientific' model of biomedical risk was present in all of the women's discourse. Women who chose Caesareans were however most committed to a technocratic model of birth and constructed the choice to have a Caesarean in terms of biomedical risk management. As in other studies, women choosing Caesarean sections constructed them as a 'safer choice' (for example Bryant et al. 2007, Fenwick et al. 2010, Douché and Carryer 2011). Women who chose to give birth at home had conflicting positions on the technocratic risk discourse, veering between compliance and resistance (see also Klassen 2001). Thus, while women who had Caesarean births fully invested in biomedical constructions of risk, women who gave birth at home were active in constructing an alternative that emphasised the relational, knowing and capable birthing body over biomedical definitions of risk.

While biomedical risk is often assumed to be the only form of risk salient to women in relation to childbirth (see Hausman 2005, Possamai-Inesedy 2006, Seibold et al. 2010), this study showed that women are rendered doubly risky in relation to childbirth. They are classified by biomedical discourse as bodies at risk of complication, abnormality and death but are also positioned as vulnerable bodies at risk of exposure, loss of dignity and objectification, particularly in medicalised settings. Women thus have to negotiate the doubly risky embodiment of childbirth, in terms of both biomedical risks and the emotional risks of potentially losing bodily control, dignity and privacy during the intensely embodied birth experience.

Women who chose Caesarean sections escaped the embodied birth experience and its threats to bodily integrity through surgical birth. Women who gave birth at home resisted the definition of birthing bodies as inherently threatening and instead constructed birthing embodiment as a risky situation only in medicalised hospital settings. They constructed the birthing body as vulnerable to objectification, loss of dignity and shaming in biomedical and technocratic contexts (see also Lyerly 2006). While the dominance of biomedical definitions of risk in relation to birth have been confirmed by other studies (for example Possamai-Inesedy 2006, Miller and Shriver 2012), the birthing body as itself a site of risk for women has not been widely recognised. This neglected aspect of risk was found to be central to women's meaning-making about risk and birth. Furthermore, women's birth choices were found to function as strategies aimed at minimising the potential vulnerabilities and risks of birthing embodiment (shaming, loss of dignity and objectification).

Women who chose to give birth at home, as in other studies (see Miller and Shriver 2012; Lindgren *et al.* 2008; Edwards and Murphy-Lawless 2006; and Viisainen 2000), constructed complex and alternative definitions of risk in relation to childbirth. Furthermore, they were engaged in a process of developing an alternative approach to childbirth emphasising connection and bodily knowing over biomedical constructions of risk. Our findings support those of Klassen (2001); Cheyney (2008, 2011) and Macdonald (2006), which showed the subversive and 'systems-challenging' (Cheyney 2008) potentialities of the knowledge constructed by women who chose to give birth at home.

In this article we show the contradictions inherent in women's negotiations of risk in relation to birth. While a 'technico-scientific' model of biomedical risk was present as an over-arching interpretative framework for all of the women, in their talk about making everyday birth choices, risks pertaining to the treatment of the birthing body were also evident. The meanings accorded to risk in relation to birth thus emerged as multiple and were not confined to biomedical meanings. Furthermore, in their accounts of the lived experience of home birth, women challenged biomedical meanings of risk by constructing an alternative approach to birth based on concrete, relational and embodied forms of knowing. This confirms the importance of 'situated rationalities' (Tulloch and Lupton 2003, p. 9) or lay risk knowledge (such as intuition) over expert knowledge in everyday lived experience. When describing their bodily, lived birth experiences, home birth was not defined in relation to biomedical risk but emerged as a transcendent and empowering activity and source of relational and embodied knowledge for women who gave birth at home. We can see the ways in which the choice to birth at home (always a negative risk in biomedical discourse) emerges not only as an issue of safety and negative biomedical risk but also as a positive potentiality (Tulloch and Lupon 2003). Furthermore, in affirming the capable, trustworthy and knowing body of birth, these women destabilised narrow biomedical constructions of risk and childbirth.

This study suggests that biomedical models of risk in relation to birth were important for middle-class women in South Africa. In line with findings in other developing world contexts such as Mexico (Smith-Oka 2012) and Ghana (Denham 2012), we found that biomedical definitions of risk are increasingly authoritative in relation to birth. In contrast to other studies, we found that the vulnerabilities and risks of birthing embodiment (potential objectification, loss of dignity and shaming) in biomedical contexts emerged as a central element of risk for women. It is not clear to what extent this aspect of risk and birth is specific to the context of middle-class birth in South Africa. Studies such as Bradby's (1998), based on interviews with rural women in Bolivia, suggest that the risks of medicalised birth, in terms of potential lack of privacy, lack of respect for bodily integrity and non-dignified care, might be an important issue for women in other contexts. Further research is needed to explore the meanings and implications of the embodied vulnerabilities and risks of medicalised birth for women in different settings.

The findings of this study are based on a relatively small sample of women in the South African context who defined their home birth and Caesarean section as self-chosen. These findings therefore do not necessarily reflect the experience of women who choose home birth or elective Caesarean section in other contexts. The research is also limited in its focus on predominantly middle-class, white women. More research is needed in the South African context (and internationally) with women of different socio-economic and racial backgrounds to explore risk constructions more broadly and in relation to material realities of deprivation and lack of birth choices. The study is further limited in its reliance upon risk theories emanating from developed world settings.

Conclusion

In this article we have shown the complex constructions of risk in women's discourse about choosing to birth either at home or via an elective Caesarean section. Expert knowledge and biomedical definitions of risk served as over-arching interpretative frameworks in which women negotiated the uncertainties of birth. Women who chose to give birth at home however constructed situated and embodied knowledges of childbirth that challenged expert, technocratic risk definitions. Our data confirm the complexities of 'situated rationalities' (Tulloch and Lupton 2003, p. 9) in relation to risk constructions. It also points to the salience of other forms of bodily risk (see Chadwick and Foster 2013) such as body objectification, shaming and loss of dignity for women in relation to childbirth.

References

Annandale, E., 1988. How midwives accomplish natural birth: managing risk and balancing expectation. *Social problems*, 35 (2), 95–110.

Beck, U., 1992. *Risk society: towards a new modernity*. London: Sage.

Bogg, L., *et al.*, 2010. Dramatic increase of Cesarean deliveries in the midst of health reforms in rural China. *Social science & medicine*, 70, 1544–1549.

Boucher, D., *et al.*, 2009. Staying home to give birth: why women in the United States choose home birth. *Journal of midwifery & women's health*, 54, 119–126.

Bourdieu, P., 2005. Habitus. *In*: J. Hillier and E. Rooksby, eds. *Habitus: a sense of place*. Aldershot: Ashgate, 43–52.

Bradby, B., 1998. Like a video: the sexualisation of childbirth in Bolivia. *Reproductive health matters*, 6 (12), 50–56.

Bryant, J., *et al.*, 2007. Caesarean birth: consumption, safety, order and good mothering. *Social science & medicine*, 65, 1192–1201.

Chadwick, R. and Foster, D., 2013. Technologies of gender and childbirth choices: home birth, elective caesarean and white femininities in South Africa. *Feminism & psychology*, 23 (3), 317–338.

Cheyney, M., 2008. Homebirth as systems-challenging praxis: knowledge, power, and intimacy in the birthplace. *Qualitative health research*, 18, 254–267.

Cheyney, M., 2011. Reinscribing the birthing body: homebirth as ritual performance. *Medical anthropology quarterly*, 25 (4), 519–542.

Davis-Floyd, R., 2003. *Birth as an American rite of passage*. Berkeley, CA: University of California Press.

Davis-Floyd, R. and Sargent, C., eds., 1997. *Childbirth and authoritative knowledge: cross-cultural perspectives*. Berkeley, CA: University of California Press.

Denham, A., 2012. Shifting maternal responsibilities and the trajectory of blame in northern Ghana. *In*: L. Fordyce and A. Maraesa, eds. *Risk, reproduction, and narratives of experience*. Nashville, TN: Vanderbilt University Press, 173–189.

Diniz, S. and Chacham, A., 2004. 'The cut above' and 'the cut below': the abuse of caesareans and episiotomy in São Paulo, Brazil. *Reproductive health matters*, 12, 100–110.

Douché, J. and Carryer, J., 2011. Caesarean section in the absence of need: a pathologising paradox for public health? *Nursing inquiry*, 18 (2), 143–153.

Edwards, N., 2005. *Birthing autonomy: women's experiences of planning home births.* London: Routledge.

Edwards, N. and Murphy-Lawless, J., 2006. The instability of risk: women's perspectives on risk and safety in childbirth. *In*: A. Symon, ed. *Risk and choice in maternity care: an international perspective.* Philadelphia, PA: Elsevier/Churchill Livingstone, 35–50.

Fenwick, J., Staff, L., and Creedy, D., 2010. Why do women request caesarean section in a normal, healthy first pregnancy? *Midwifery*, 26, 394–400.

Fox, B. and Worts, D., 1999. Revisiting the critique of medicalized childbirth: a contribution to the sociology of birth. *Gender & society*, 13 (3), 326–346.

Grosz, E., 1989. *Sexual subversions: three French feminists.* Sydney: Allen & Unwin.

Hausman, B., 2005. Risky business: framing childbirth in hospital settings. *Journal of medical humanities*, 26 (1), 23–38.

Helén, I., 2004. Technics over life: risk, ethics and the existential condition in high-tech antenatal care. *Economy & society*, 33 (1), 28–51.

Jordan, B., 1997. Authoritative knowledge and its construction. *In*: R. Davis-Floyd and C. Sargent, eds. *Childbirth and authoritative knowledge: cross-cultural perspectives.* Berkeley, CA: University of California Press, 55–79.

Karlström, A., *et al.*, 2011. Behind the myth – few women prefer caesarean section in the absence of obstetrical factors. *Midwifery*, 27 (5), 620–627.

Kelhä, M., 2009. Too old to become a mother? Risk constructions in 35+ women's experiences of pregnancy, child-birth, and postnatal care. *Nordic journal of feminist & gender research*, 17 (2), 89–103.

Kingdon, C., *et al.*, 2003. Who's choosing caesarean section? *British journal of midwifery*, 11 (6), 391.

Klassen, P., 2001. *Blessed events: religion and home birth in America.* Princeton University Press.

Knaak, S., 2010. Contextualising risk, constructing choice: breastfeeding and good mothering in risk society. *Health, risk & society*, 12 (4), 369–383.

Kornelsen, J., 2005. Essences and imperatives: an investigation of technology in childbirth. *Social science & medicine*, 61, 1495–1504.

Lankshear, G., Ettore, E., and Mason, D., 2005. Decision-making, uncertainty and risk: exploring the complexity of work processes in NHS delivery suites. *Health, risk & society*, 7 (4), 361–377.

Law, J., 2000. The politics of breastfeeding: assessing risk, dividing labor. *Signs*, 25 (2), 407–450.

Lawrie, T., de Jager, M., and Hofmeyr, J., 2001. High cesarean section rates for pregnant medical practitioners in South Africa. *International journal of gynecology & obstetrics*, 72 (1), 71–73.

Lee, E., 2007a. Health, morality and infant feeding: British mothers experiences of formula milk use in the early weeks. *Sociology of health & illness*, 29 (7), 1075–1090.

Lee, E., 2007b. Infant feeding in risk society. *Health, risk & society*, 9 (3), 295–309.

Lee, E., 2008. Living with risk in the age of 'intensive motherhood': maternal identity and infant feeding. *Health, risk & society*, 10 (5), 467–477.

Lindgren, H., *et al.*, 2008. Perceptions of risk and risk management among 735 women who opted for a home birth. *Midwifery*, 26, 163–172.

Lupton, D., 1999a. *Risk.* London: Routledge.

Lupton, D. ed., 1999b. *Risk and sociocultural theory.* Cambridge University Press.

Lupton, D., ed., 1999c. Risk and the ontology of pregnant embodiment. *In Risk and sociocultural theory.* Cambridge University Press, 59–85.

Lupton, D., 2008. You feel so responsible': australian mothers' concepts and experiences related to promoting the health and development of their young children. *In*: H. Zoller and M. Dutta, eds. *Emerging perspectives in health communication: meaning, culture, and power.* New York: Routledge, 113–128.

Lupton, D., 2011. 'The best thing for the baby': mothers' concepts and experiences related to promoting their infants' health and development. *Health, risk & society*, 13 (7–8), 637–651.

Lupton, D., 2012. 'Precious cargo': foetal subjects, risk and reproductive citizenship. *Critical public health*, 22 (3), 329–340.

Lupton, D. and Tulloch, J., 1998. The adolescent 'unfinished body': reflexivity and HIV/AIDS risk. *Body & society*, 4 (2), 19–34.

Lupton, D. and Tulloch, J., 2002a. 'Life would be pretty dull without risk': voluntary risk-taking and its pleasures. *Health, risk & society*, 4 (2), 113–124.

Lupton, D. and Tulloch, J., 2002b. Risk is part of your life': risk epistemologies among a group of Australians. *Sociology*, 36 (2), 317–334.

Lyerly, A., 2006. Shame, gender, birth. *Hypatia*, 21 (1), 101–118.

Macdonald, M., 2006. Gender expectations: natural bodies and natural births in the new midwifery in Canada. *Medical anthropology quarterly*, 20 (2), 235–256.

Mackenzie Bryers, H. and van Teijlingen, E., 2010. Risk, theory, social and medical models: a critical analysis of the concept of risk in maternity care. *Midwifery*, 26 (5), 488–496.

Martin, E., 1987. *The woman in the body: a cultural analysis of reproduction*. Milton Keynes: Open University Press.

McCourt, C., Bick, D., and Weaver, J., 2004. Caesarean section: perceived demand. *British journal of midwifery*, 12 (7), 412–413.

McDonald, K., Amir, L., and Davey, M., 2011. Maternal bodies and medicines: a commentary on risk and decision-making of pregnant and breastfeeding women and health professionals. *BMC public health*, 11 (5), S5.

Miller, A. and Shriver, T., 2012. Women's childbirth preferences and practices in the United States. *Social science & medicine*, 75, 709–716.

Munro, S., Kornelsen, J., and Hutton, E., 2009. Decision-making in patient-initiated elective cesarean delivery: the influence of birth stories. *Journal of midwifery & women's health*, 54 (4), 373–379.

Murphy, E., 2003. Expertise and forms of knowledge in the government of families. *Sociology of health & illness*, 51 (4), 433–462.

Murphy, E., 2004. Risk, maternal ideologies, and infant feeding. *In*: J. Germov and L. Williams, eds. *A sociology of food and nutrition*. Oxford University Press, 242–258.

Naidoo, N. and Moodley, J., 2009. Rising rates of caesarean sections: an audit of caesarean sections in specialist private practice. *South African family practice*, 51 (3), 254–258.

Parker, I., 1992. *Discourse dynamics: critical analysis for social and individual psychology*. London: Routledge.

Possamai-Inesedy, A., 2006. Confining risk: choice and responsibility in childbirth in a risk society. *Health sociology review*, 15, 406–414.

Potter, J., 1997. Discourse and critical social psychology. *In*: T. Ibanez and L. Iniguez, eds. *Critical social psychology*. London: Sage, 55–66.

Root, R. and Browner, C., 2001. Practices of the pregnant self: compliance with and resistance to prenatal norms. *Culture, medicine & psychiatry*, 25, 195–223.

Rothberg, A. and Macleod, H., 2005. Private-sector caesarean sections in perspective. *South African medical journal*, 95 (4), 257–260.

Rothman, B., 1982. *In labor: women and power in the birthplace*. New York: W.W. Norton & Company.

Ruhl, L., 1999. Liberal governance and prenatal care: risk and regulation in pregnancy. *Economy & society*, 28 (1), 95–117.

Scamell, M., 2011. The swan effect in midwifery talk and practice: a tension between normality and the language of risk. *Sociology of health & illness*, 33 (7), 987–1001.

Scamell, M. and Alaszewski, A., 2012. Fateful moments and the categorisation of risk: midwifery practice and the ever-narrowing window of normality during childbirth. *Health, risk & society*, 14 (2), 207–221.

Seibold, C., et al., 2010. 'Lending the space': midwives perceptions of birth space and clinical risk management. *Midwifery*, 26, 526–531.

Smith-Oka, V., 2012. Bodies of risk: constructing motherhood in a Mexican public hospital. *Social science and medicine*, 75, 2275–2282.

Smith, V., Devane, D., and Murphy-Lawless, J., 2012. Risk in maternity care: a concept analysis. *International journal of childbirth*, 2 (2), 126–135.

South African Demographic and Health Survey. 2003, 2007. *Department of Health, Medical Research Council*. Pretoria: Department of Health.

Tshibangu, K., et al., 2002. Incidence and outcome of caesarean section in the private sector – 3-year experience at Pretoria Gynaecological Hospital. *South African medical journal*, 92 (12), 956–959.

Tulloch, J. and Lupton, D. eds., 2003. *Risk and everyday life*. London: Sage.

Viisainen, K., 2000. The moral dangers of home birth: parents' perceptions of risks in home birth in Finland. *Sociology of health & illness*, 22 (6), 792–814.

Pluralist risk cultures: the sociology of childbirth in Vanuatu

Karen Lane

Faculty of Arts and Education, School of Humanities and Social Sciences, Deakin University, Melbourne, Victoria, Australia

Western medical approaches to childbirth typically locate risk in women's bodies, making it axiomatic that 'good' maternity care is associated with medically trained attendants. This logic has been extrapolated to developing societies, like Vanuatu, an Island state in the Pacific, struggling to provide good maternity care in line with the World Health Organization's Millennium Development Goals. These goals include the reduction of maternal mortality by two-thirds by 2015, but Vanuatu must overcome challenging hurdles – medical, social and environmental – to achieve this goal. Vanuatu is a hybridised society: one where the pre-modern and modern coincide in parallel institutions, processes and practices. In 2010, I undertook an inductive study of 30 respondents from four main subcultures – women living in outer rural communities with limited access to Western-trained health workers; women from inner urban communities with ease of access to medical clinics; traditional birth attendants who are formally untrained but highly specialised and practised mainly in remote communities; and Western-trained medical clinicians (obstetricians and midwives). I invited all the participants to comment on what constituted a 'good birth'. In this article, I show that participants interpreted this variously according to how they believed the uncertainties of childbirth could be managed. Objectivist approaches that define risk as an objective reality amenable to quantifiable measurement are thus rendered inadequate. Interpretivist approaches better explain the reality that social actors not only find risk in different sites but gravitate towards different practices, discourses and individuals they can trust especially those with whom they feel a strong sense of community. Strategies are, therefore, formed less through scientific rationality but according to feelings and emotions and the lived experience. The concept of risk cultures conveys this complexity; they are formed around *values* rather than calculable rationalities. Risk cultures form self-reflexively to manage contingent circumstances.

Introduction

In this article, I draw on findings from an inductive qualitative study conducted in 2010 comprising 30 respondents. In this study, I examined how different groups with diverse interpretive lens and in the context of hybrid pre-modern and modern knowledge traditions and cultures as well as challenging local exigencies – social, economic and geographical – talked about the achievement of a 'good birth'. Like professional clinicians and pregnant women in high-income countries who have been assimilated into a normative risk culture surrounding birth (Coxon, Scamell, & Alaszewski, 2012), all groups expressed their views in terms of how to manage hazards, uncertainty and risk; the latter was discussed in terms of how to avoid unknown, negative contingencies that they associated with birth (Lupton, 2013a). It was never a matter of a straightforward safe event for all respondents. A risk consciousness had developed in Vanuatu (Lupton, 2013a; Rothman, 2014), although it is well to bear in mind that negative outcomes in childbirth in developing economies are more prevalent than in developed regimes. That is, rates of infant and maternal mortality are visibly higher, medical resources and transport are less available and the economic capacities of women are meagre. Nonetheless, what constitutes risk for ni-Vanuatu actors (i.e. citizens of Vanuatu) and therefore how to manage it remained contentious. In this article, I draw on these data to consider the different ways in which risk is constructed in the context of childbirth and the different strategies individuals use to manage the uncertainties of childbirth in Vanuatu.

Uncertainty, risk and childbirth in developing countries

Most social scientists accept that risk is shaped by social contexts. For example, Heyman, Alaszewski, and Brown (2012) argue that it can be seen as a metaphor signifying 'a culturally manufactured lens which shapes perceptions' (p. 107). Such an approach is a critique of objectivist approaches such as The Royal Society Risk Working Group definition in which risk is defined as an objective reality that is amenable to quantifiable measurement, namely:

> the probability (3) that a particular adverse (2) event (1) occurs during a stated period of time (4a) or results from a particular challenge (4b). As a probability in the sense of statistical theory risk obeys all the formal laws of combined probabilities. (1992, p. 2)

As Heyman et al. (2012) point out, all components of this definition are open to social interpretation. Indeed, much of the social science literature on risk is grounded in the interpretivist understanding that reality is the outcome of active interpretation by social actors with multifaceted biographies shaped by complex forces. As Zinn (2008) notes, debates about risk thus need to be considered within social, political, historical, economic and cultural contexts. Objectivist (positivist) theories of risk (and knowledge) that posit risks are amenable to calculable rational measurement making them predictable and preventable (Alaszewski & Burgess, 2007; Green, 1999) are challenged by social constructionist (interpretivist) theories of risk (and knowledge) (Rothfield, 1995). In these social constructionist theories, risk is defined as a contingent, unknown and negative outcome; its negativity implies risk is inherently normative (Lupton, 2013a). It is not that positivist methodologies (such as the randomised controlled trial) produce redundant information but they fail to acknowledge, as constructionist methodologies show, the contested nature of what frames and constitutes risk objects. Those using the constructionist approach begin with the proposition that all knowledge claims (including risk) are informed by individualised cognition and affective responses to social and contextual forces (Lupton, 2013b). Constructionism is able to embrace the idea that risk is contingent, unpredictable and variously interpreted (Turner, 2014).

Within the social sciences, debates about risk have developed and intensified, indicating endemic philosophical, disciplinary and administrative complexities. Beck originally raised the debate about the generic risks of modernisation where the distribution of 'bads' comes to be felt by everyone (Beck, 1992), and although he failed to define risk adequately, his thesis stimulated vigorous debate about a number of issues. One relates to the ways in which negative outcomes in the future needed to be contextualised within definite historical, political, cultural and economic circumstances. Another issue relates to the ways in which risks are delineated from hazards; the latter are current and detectable (although diversely interpreted) while risks comprise negative consequences in the future that may well be 'contingent, uncertain and unpredictable' (Turner, 2014, p. 12). A further issue relates to the ways in which risks relate to outcomes that are unpredictable in terms of when they may emerge, who will bear the full brunt of them if they occur, how those affected will perceive them and how they are managed. It follows that governments may lack the political machinery to adequately manage risks, especially those that occur without their knowledge or consent. Such risks would include the risks of uneven and unregulated economic development and global trading inequalities (Turner, 2014), as well as the risks of climate change and modernist science and technologies (Beck, 1992, 2009).

Risk has also been an organising trope of all societies, pre-modern, modern and late modern/postmodern in the sense that it has been used to explicate social events and to authorise certain forms of social organisation to manage it. In pre-modern societies, misfortune was explained in terms of transgressing social and/or religious rules and mores (Alaszewski, 2003, 2015; Douglas, 1992; Douglas & Wildavsky, 1982). In modern societies characterised by secularisation, industrialisation and urbanisation, the gathering of information into statistical categories via the scientific method represents an attempt 'to tame chance' (Hacking, 1990); to explain causation in terms of tangible, manageable and predictable entities rather than mystical tyrannical forces. In modern societies, organised risk management regimes produce risks that are managed through the welfare state, centralised surveillance mechanisms, like hospitalisation, mass screenings, mass vaccinations and transfer payments. In neoliberal regimes, Crook (1999) calls attention to 'the overproduction and undercontrol of risks' (Crook, 1999, 180); new health disciplines and citizens become vectors of risk management so interpretations of what constitutes a risk object become multiplied (Crook, 1999; Dean, 1999).

Medicalisation and the management of risk

The governmentality theorists of risk and risk management (e.g. Crook, 1999; Dean, 1999) drew on Foucault's thesis that the practice of medicine that emerged in Western regimes in the late eighteenth and nineteenth centuries adopted the scientific method to gain a competitive advantage over other healing practices aided (Foucault, 1975). Via state sanction of administrative and legal infrastructures, medical professions secured a market monopoly that established medical codified knowledge as authoritative knowledge while simultaneously casting contenders as quacks, witches and unscientific imposters (Lane, 2006; Murphy-Lawless, 1998). Medical professionalisation continued to fortify a medical hierarchy by enacting the cultural work of 'a labour of division' (Abbott, 1988; Allen, 2002; Fournier, 2000; Lane, 2012); a privileged boundary around its sphere of practice. Later developments led to the emergence of disciplinary offshoots such as medical epidemiology that weighted complex variables in determining future adverse possibilities and how to avoid them. By the 1980s, evidence-based medicine (EBM) emerged to remove decision-making from limited practitioner evidence and idiosyncrasy towards a more robust scientific base. It also secured informed consent (Heyman et al., 2012). By the end of the twentieth century, economic and political crises on a global scale had ushered in a new era of neoliberalism (Tonkiss, 2006) accompanied by new strategies of governance to better contain a burgeoning health budget. Midwifery, for example, was seen to offer good risk management in the birthplace bringing to partial fruition midwifery's long-term challenges to the medical hierarchy since professionalisation in the nineteenth century. In a parallel way, nurse-practitioners emerged to partially undertake some of the more routine tasks of medical practice (Lane, 2006).

When modernist governments commissioned medicine from the late nineteenth century to manage the health of citizens in pursuit of the future wealth of the nation, professionalisation medical practitioners framed adverse events around the concept of risk, rather than sin or moral retribution (Alaszewski 2003, in press; Turner, 2014).

The emergent normative consciousness of birth-as-risk dovetailed with concurrent social and political shifts, namely the link between first-wave feminism and scientific mothering underpinned by maternalist ideologies. Importantly, scientific motherhood not only imposed the burden of the health of families and nation on women but at the same time rendered them incapable of doing so and thus keenly motivated to seek reliable advice. Further, in their search for relief of the acute pain of childbirth, women played an active part in welcoming the interventions of obstetric science (Reisman, 1983; Rothman, 2014), confirming its 'perceptions of effectiveness' (Hallgrimsdottir & Benner, 2014). When the twinning of good health and responsible citizenship heralded the new public health movement, the medical gaze turned to childbirth, cementing the ascendancy of obstetrics in the management of childbirth which was, by now, marked with the indelible nature of risk.

For their part, governments, both modernist and then neoliberal, institutionalised the notion of childbirth-as-risk because governments harbour 'dreams of order' (Crook, 1999; Dean, 1999; Foucault, 1975) and sanctioned various arrangements to contain it. Auditing of organisational outcomes and processes was one effect (Power, 1997). Medicalisation was another; everyday life becomes medicalised (Alaszewski, in press; Chadwick & Foster, 2014; Scamell & Alaszewski, 2012), including and especially birth as a major plank in the management of risks to the individual, to families, to the workforce and to the nation's future gross domestic product. Legal arrangements protecting medical monopolies express the expectation that medicine successfully contains risk. Medical negligence legislation enforces this premise disciplining medical practitioners to avoid what the medical canon regards as the inherent risks of the body. The effect is the institutionalisation of defensive medicine achieved through a raft of disciplinary technologies governing medical practice while assigning other, contesting modalities to subordinate status, like midwifery. Midwives are made workplace-compliant by machinery such as spheres of practice, protocols and practice guidelines presided over by professional associations and legalities. Over time other administrative measures are imposed on populations to manage uncertain futures such as screening programmes, mass vaccinations and centralised hospital care for childbirth. Under neoliberal regimes facing budget crises and the globalisation of health risks, individuals are recruited to manage their own lifestyle behaviours and decision-making (Crook, 1999; Lupton, 2013a). Individuals become self-reflexive about managing risk (Beck, 1992; Lash, 2000; Lash, Giddens, & Beck, 1994) as welfare state programmes are cut, medical disasters and media coverage of medical negligence cases erode trust in medical expertise (Alaszewski, 2003) and as Western societies deal with the exponential rise of chronic illnesses.

The reality is that chance can never be tamed (Hacking, 1990) and the 'dreams of order' will always fail (Crook, 1999), although the rise of an audit culture (Power, 1997) signifies continuing efforts to predict and manage risks. The randomised control trial becomes the optimal tool at the heart of EBM. However, childbirth is an especially fraught area of health care because birth has also been medicalised. In approaching their 'fateful moment' (Scamell & Alaszewski, 2012), women are not only chronically naive about outcomes, they approach the experience with a sense of foreboding about what has become medically framed as an inherently dangerous business. From a biomedical, objectivist approach (Rothfield, 1995), birth is dangerous because the body is fragile. Midwives adopting a social model of birth premised on achieving safe outcomes through good social supports, on the other hand, are much more confident about the ability of the female body to deliver a baby safely. Yet midwives remain watchful because risks hover on the horizon: they espouse normality but their practice is disciplined by biomedical risk discourses and institutional protocols (Scamell & Alaszewski, 2012). Women in developed societies facing decisions about birth thus confront oppositional paradigms on the body and birth. Women in developing societies confront yet another – the clash between pre-modern, traditional cultures of birth and an imported Western model. How they negotiate these schisms depends upon the social location of the beholder (Lupton, 2013a; Shilling, 2003; Turner, 2014).

The fear of an adverse outcome engenders various strategies such as the cultivation of trust in order to avoid risks; strategies that occur at macro-, meso- and micro-interactional levels (Dibben & Lean, 2003). For example, women in advanced Western regimes are more likely to trust expert systems (Lash et al., 1994), reflected in the move by 99.4% of women to birth in hospital. Conversely, they eschew home birth despite equivalent rates of safety because the biomedical paradigm represents a dominant discourse (Coxon, Sandall, & Fulop, 2014). However, their implicit faith in the expert system of medicalised birth is somewhat misplaced. Hospital birth in the West has been accompanied by increasing rates of caesarean section (30–35%), despite WHO advice that a caesarean section rate of 10–15% is the ceiling rate for developed nations comprising generations of healthy women who also attract high rates of other surgical interventions. Marsden Wagner (1994, 2001), a senior obstetrician, has been an outspoken critic of such routine medical interventions claiming that centralised hospital birth with its loss of autonomy for women has few compensatory benefits. In fact, in the US (a developed nation with high caesarean section rates), maternal mortality rates continue to rise annually (Creanga et al., 2015) and many US women are disappointed with the experience (Declercq & Chalmers, 2008). (It should be noted that 91% Scottish women rated their care as excellent but this related to number of carers; Cheyne, Skar, Peterson, David, & Hodgkiss, 2013.) The point is that the Western biomedical model with its reductionist and objectifying philosophy of care (Grosz, 1994; Shilling, 2003) and centralised organisational model is non-optimal for many women in developing economies, especially remote area women. Yet developing countries like Vanuatu are embracing a Western model of birth when the conditions and challenges they face are entirely different.

Risk and birth in Vanuatu

Birth and risks in developing economies

In Third World regimes, almost two-thirds of births occur at home and only half are attended by a trained birth attendant (WHO, 1996). Providing skilled care has become a critical point of intervention because of the 300,000–400,000 maternal deaths per annum worldwide. More than 50% occur in only six countries (India, Nigeria, Pakistan, Afghanistan, Ethiopia and the Democratic Republic of the Congo); all are war-torn countries, except for India (Bhutta et al., 2010). Deaths occur primarily in the first two days after birth (Hurt & Ronsmans, 2002; Ronsmans & Graham, 2006). The majority (80%) are due to bleeding (haemorrhage), infection, complications following unsafe abortion, eclampsia and obstructed labour. Around 10–20 million women suffer physical or mental morbidities due to poor childbirth management (Ashford, 2014; Murray & Lopez, 1998) and many extend to the long term. To remedy the serious shortfall in good maternity care, the standard approach is to train many more skilled attendants – around 400,000 midwives need to be trained to cover the 45–60 million births per annum currently unattended by any health professional (Byrne & Morgan, 2011; Walraven & Weeks, 1999). Also, in poor remote regions women lack access to quality care because their health is not prioritised, warning signs of complications go unrecognised and women fear the costs of care or deficient care from health facilities (Ashford, 2014).

In addressing these problems, traditional birth attendants were trained in the 1970s to attend home births and thus reduce neonatal deaths (aged 0–27 days) that account for 41% (3575 million) of all deaths in children younger than 5 years. But in the 1990s, a Western medical system was introduced and traditional birth attendants became redundant. The new regime prioritised rational technical knowledge, medical technologies and centralised hospital birth, together with a system of regional health posts staffed by trained health workers (Ensor & Cooper, 2004; Hoj, Da Silva, Hedegaard, Sandstrom, & Aaby, 2003; Lassi, Haider, & Bhutta, 2010; Ray & Salihu, 2004). The decision to relinquish traditional birth attendants meant their localised cultural knowledge, tacit skills and years of expertise were lost. Women no longer had a known carer, and the decision was based on false premises. Baseline data were missing in the 1970s (Kruske & Barclay, 2004), so the charge that they had failed to reduce infant and maternal mortality rates was founded on inadequate data. Further, a Western health model is not always suited to local conditions. In Vanuatu, for example, problems are steeped in wider infrastructural deficits including poverty, poor nutrition, illiteracy and lack of information regarding fertility control, lack of emergency obstetric procedures, inadequate transport and inadequate linkages between health centres and communities. By contrast, community-based interventions (including traditional attendants) have indicated good outcomes. In short, judgements of the efficacy of traditional attendants that failed to factor in social context, culture, history and values led to a precipitous dismissal of a strategy that could bridge gaps in remote and regional communities (Lassi et al., 2010; Sibley, Sipe, & Koblinsky, 2004).

Adherence to Western medical techniques has brought its own problems. Vanuatu midwives, for example, have been trained to instruct women to lie passively to give birth, they apply pressure on the perineum and cord to aid expulsion of the placenta and they ignore villagers' cultural and spiritual values. Often women birth alone because relatives are banned from the birth room (Barclay, 1997; Lane, 2013). Biomedical theories of the body and birth are, therefore, objectifying and reductionist: they concentrate on biology but ignore biography and context. As a simple monocausal model, clinicians accept as a realist ontological given that patients signify imminently emergent pathologies. Isolated from a social and historical context, women's bodies are constructed as primary sites of risk, but many developing countries have complex historical, social, cultural and geographical barriers that need to be inserted into the causal matrix of risk factors. Such factors are discussed below in the case of Vanuatu.

Vanuatu: a geographical, economic and cultural overview

Vanuatu is described as a stable, upper-middle income country located in Oceania (Quandl, 2013; World Bank, 2013) in the South Pacific. Other indicators point to a small and fragile social structure with a skewed population living mainly in rural areas (74.78%). First inhabited by Melanesians, now 80% of the population lives in rural, isolated villages growing their own food supplies. Primary education is mandatory; the adult literacy rate is 82.57%. As an indicator of globalisation, in 2008 of the total population of 218,519 (World Statistics) a mere 7.8% used the Internet.

The external physical environment presents multiple risk factors. The islands are steep with unstable soils and a paucity of freshwater. Only 9% of the land can be used for growing permanent crops. Population growth at 2.4% a year exerts pressure on land and resources needed for agriculture, grazing, hunting and fishing. Fish stocks are being depleted and islands deforested through logging of high-value timber and much arable land is being converted to coconut and cattle export markets. Since the majority of Vanuatu's population (78.5%) lives in isolated rural areas with negligible access to markets or employment, Vanuatu citizens are locked into subsistence economies. The 21.5% of the population who live either in Port Vila (15.7%) or in Luganville (5.8%) and who typically work in the tourist industry receive meagre profits largely repatriated to foreign owners. Life expectancy is 71 years, and 8.5% of the population is reportedly undernourished. Traditional values and authority structures are increasingly attenuated in urban villages (Peace Corps Vanuatu, 2013), leading to a rise in the incidence of young single mothers devoid of familial support or support from the father. Both rural and urban populations face considerable challenges in achieving good health outcomes. Most have incomes within the lowest quintile while social welfare services, including health care, remain minimal although churches and non-government organisations (NGOs) provide some support.

To meet these difficulties, two parallel systems of health care have emerged. Sometimes, they clash, causing disagreement among actors about the site of risk. The formal system (Bryers & van Teijlingen, 2010; Pickstone & Cooter, 2000) is a centralised Western medical model; risk is located primarily within the body. The second, informal system is delivered by traditional healers using bush medicines; villagers often attribute risk to social transgressions. They also appeal to higher spiritual forces, either a Christian god or animism, to resolve problems. At the national level, a comprehensive reproductive health programme has been put into place. It is supported by the UN Population Fund and other stakeholders around family planning/contraception including widespread distribution of condoms, the morning after pill, IUD insertion and Deprovera injections available at local health sites designed to modernise the health system. In addition, educational programmes target HIV/AIDS, cervical cancer and domestic violence/gender issues. Modest levels of health expenditure ($US190.66 per capita/per annum) funds minimal health professionals: 2.35 nurses per 1000 people and only 0.1 physicians per 1000 population. Maternal mortality rates and infant mortality rates (WHO, 1997) are key indicators of global health inequalities putting Vanuatu in the middle of the range with a maternal mortality rate of 86/100,000 deaths a year and infant mortality rate of 11.40 deaths/live births in 2013. (This may be compared to a developed nation like Australia with a low maternal mortality rate (.006 deaths/1000 births) and low infant mortality rate (0.049/1000 births) (World Bank, 2013)). Vanuatu's mid-range maternity risk status (on a global scale) allows researchers of maternity care to appreciate typical problems facing so-called upper-income developing economies with sizable geographical and economic barriers as they attempt to meet the accelerated Millennium Development Goals 3, 4 and 5 relating to the empowerment of women and girls. This includes significant reductions in infant and maternal mortality rates.

Maternity services in Vanuatu

Between one half and two-thirds of women experience limited access to biomedical maternity services (WHO, 1997). In 2010, there were two obstetricians at the Pt Vila Hospital and two others serving the entire population (218,519) scattered among 82 islands of volcanic origin (65 of them inhabited) with about 800 miles (1300 km) between the islands in the north and those in the south. Vanuatu health services are widely distributed, but they remain sparsely available and accessed by rural and remote village women only by foot. For example, there are four levels of health services dealing with maternity issues: aid posts staffed by a health worker; dispensaries/clinics staffed by a registered nurse; health centres (around 25 across 82 islands) staffed by a registered nurse and midwife; and four hospitals at Luganville, Tacea, Santo and Pt Vila staffed by midwives. One senior obstetrician, a junior obstetrician and two registrars are based only in hospitals where women are encouraged to attend for antenatal and delivery care or at their local health site. Apart from accessibility issues, the average cost of low-risk maternity care (around $A7) represents a significant burden on families engaged in a cash economy; families sell copra (dried coconut meat used to extract coconut oil) or other produce to pay for health care.

Childbirth in hybrid cultures: the case of Vanuatu

In this article, I argue that choices about where to locate risk in childbirth depend upon how an individual or group constructs birth, the body, the relationship between the body and the external environment, causes of pathology and weighting of variables (Asian-Pacific Resource and Research Centre for Women (ARROW), 2001; Graham, Bell, & Bullough, 2001; Starrs, 1997; WHO, 1992). Risks are real for those who confront them but are also created at least partially by those who have an interest in defining them, whether the interests are material, professional or altruistic. Pharmaceutical companies, medical clinicians, midwives, women, administrators and governments all have diverse interests and objectives in identifying risk(s) and harnessing different risk discourses for different ends (Bryers & van Teijlingen, 2010; Crook, 1999; Dean, 1999; Lane, 2012; Lupton, 1999; Walsh & Downe, 2004). For example, the discourse of risk has been appropriated by some obstetricians to achieve compliance from women and midwives (De Vries, Benoit, Van Teijlingen, & Wrede, 2001; Walsh, 2007), prompting critics to argue that risk ratings are used, not primarily as a safety measure for women, but for clinicians' professional interests (Lothian, 2012) and as a vehicle of social control (Foucault, 1991; Lane, 1995, 2013). Other studies find risk in the abuse and disrespect of women (Bowser & Hill, 2010), a finding echoed in research on childbirth in East Timor (Lane, 2013), while other studies locate risk in non-referral of high-risk women (Sibley et al., 2004) or in homebirth (Royal Australian and New Zealand College of Obstetricians and Gynaecologists (RANZCOG), 2011).

In this article, I examine the management of uncertainty in childbirth in a society characterised by both traditional and modern beliefs and practices where a dominant Western model is mediated by other cosmologies. Scamell and Alaszewski (2012) have argued that the window of normality in Western birthplaces is narrowed by discourses of risk systematically applied to all births despite the low probability that adverse events will occur. The risk label becomes a dominant discourse because it is sustained by a medical hierarchy. According to the canon of Western medicine, the body is fragile, women's bodies are especially fragile and the role of medicine is to intervene before things go wrong. The biomedical model is thus a fear model and an interventionist one (Lane, 1995). Tulloch and Lupton (2003) and Ostlin, Eckermann, Mishra, Nkowane, and Wallstam (2006) contend that modernisation need not precipitate technological dependency or discount women-centred models (Katz-Rothman, 1996). But where Western maternity care principles are introduced as the dominant model, the spectre of risk comes to govern birth. Yet in societies, like Vanuatu, where biomedicine competes with traditional cosmologies, healing practices and modalities, the object(s) of risk are much more diffuse and diverse. For example, the use of birth attendants is actively discouraged in line with World Health Organization (1992) recommendations and health policy on Vanuatu is to centralise births in medical facilities. But such policies have failed to extinguish customary cosmologies, technologies and practices because indigenous women and many midwives continued to recognise traditional skills and knowledge.

Or, put another way, the lens through which risk and uncertainty are viewed by the interpreter (Heyman et al., 2012; Hunt, 2003) are not only multiplied in the case of competing modalities but the biomedical lens fails to carry the same weight. In Vanuatu, for example, ritual consultation with 'the stones' resolved the dilemma of facing uncertain futures and regarded as entirely compatible with the Christian God. Imbibing of the kastom leaf for women in labour (see evidence below) and other bush medicines for other maladies can be interpreted as devices to manage uncertainties, to create social order and unity, to establish the verity of local knowledges and customs and as a corrective to Western ideas and practices surrounding birth. As Malinowksi (1922) argued, there is an instrumental rationality about these practices and a durability about them, discounting the theory of staged development that magic and religion disappear within modernity. And, as Douglas (2002) argued, the dangers that are identified selectively from a range of possible others reflect dominant discourses and arrangements. Risk is politicised (Lupton, 1999).

In this article, I examine what happens when a Western biomedical model of birth is exported to a developing economy with competing cosmologies and healing practices. In order to investigate this problematic, I posed to key actors in the ni-Vanuatu maternity system an open question, that is, how they defined a 'good birth'. Questions of risk were not used to frame the interviews to avoid the tendency to pre-empt responses or lead respondents towards interpreting birth as a risk-laden event (Henwood, Pidgeon, Sarre, Simmons, & Smith, 2008).

Methodology

In this article, I draw on data from a qualitative study of 30 social actors involved in the provision of maternity care or who were recipients of care in order to evaluate whether they perceived birth as a risk-laden event and, if so, where they located risk and how they managed it. Qualitative methods such as in-depth and non-structured interviews were most apposite to uncover this kind of rich data. Ethics clearance was obtained from Deakin University prior to the study. In 2010, the Vanuatu Ministry of Health also provided ethics clearance and issued a Letter of Introduction granting permission to the researcher to interview NGO workers, professional medical and midwifery staff and women involved in maternity services at metropolitan; provincial and central levels.

Interviews with most women were conducted in the local language with the aid of an interpreter. After the interview, the interpreter provided a full description of the evidence and this was recorded. All respondents agreed to recording of interviews.

The management of uncertainty was a second-order outcome of the primary research question that revolved around what was defined by different social actors as 'a good birth'. Only midwives/health nurses and women were interviewed at rural locations because obstetricians worked in urban-based hospitals. Traditional birth attendants were difficult to find in urban/metropolitan areas because government policy since the 1990s had phased them out, at least officially. However, they were found on the remote volcanic island of Tanna. All respondents were assured that their evidence and their identity would remain anonymous and that the researcher remained independent from government and NGOs. Respondents were not requested to provide written consent due to a general distrust of officialdom and strangers. However, verbal consent was recorded for every respondent. Where interviews were conducted in English, the researcher and interpreter compared interpretations to ensure coherence. The interpreter relayed information to the researcher immediately after the interview when respondents used the local language. The researcher worked on establishing a trusting relationship with the interpreter who was also paid a good rate for his services.

Findings

The findings from key social actors in the study are presented in terms of how they envisaged the management of uncertainty in relation to childbirth. Views relayed by women, then medical practitioners (obstetricians and midwives) and then traditional midwives are included below.

Views of mothers

Mary and Mary were both older women who each had multiple births and had recently delivered babies when I interviewed them. They lived on remote Tanna Island and during their pregnancy had consulted traditional healers and birth attendants for

> ...herbs to drink to make the baby grow and to clean the womb [and for the] kastom leaf so the baby came easily and not very painful.

Mary was aware that the doctor regarded it as '...not clean so we have to be very careful [not to tell him]'. All villagers used various herbal medicines including the kastom leaf as part of their spiritual cosmology governing the practices of everyday life:

> ...we have stones and if we need something or if someone needs to be cured we make the herbs, go to the stones and ask for help.

Traditional medicine and western medicine were both good, she claimed, because they were both given by (the Christian) God but the kastom leaf alone substantially eased labour pain, facilitated movement and, very significantly, was cost-free. Both Mary and Mary had lived on Tanna all their lives and delivered three babies at home, but they preferred hospital birth because they associated risk with unhygienic home birth practices. Another older woman, Winnie, reflecting on her four births at home and in hospital, located risk in the hospital because the midwives were negligent.

They talk a lot. There are three women there giving birth at the same time and the midwife was too busy to be with them.

Winnie explained to me that the old traditional birth attendant was safe because she observed hygienic practices, and was known and trusted, but she felt that none of the young women who had replaced her when she died were trustworthy. For one young single mother, Leviau, the village midwife was better because she was '...less expensive and not so far as the hospital'.

Woman who lived a short distance from hospital considered it to be a good option. The grandmothers in Mele (a village just outside Pt Villa) believed that hospital reduced risk because it housed all of the equipment in case something went wrong (a familiar refrain). Violet, a young mother who delivered her first baby at the Pt Vila hospital, believed that '...in the village their [meaning mothers'] lives are in danger so ... it is better to go to the hospital'. Since her own mother experienced a problem with homebirth, Violet opted for a hospital birth and stayed with relatives near Pt Vila for 1 month before her due date to attend medical checks.

For other single and married young women with experience of pregnancy and birth, Leitaki, Rose, Merilyn, Josephine and Jocelyn, risk was also located in home birth and in any birth attendant who was unknown to them, especially if the traditional attendant possessed only marginal midwifery skills. All women valued relationships with carers based upon trust and respect and were prepared to bear the considerable costs of hospital birth and the travelling time to avoid a village attendant they neither knew nor trusted. Zora, whose mother had died from a postnatal haemorrhage at home, felt safer at the hospital despite the distance. Only Leivau, a young single mother who delivered her baby at the local clinic, nominated hospital midwives directly as a site or risk: '...they were not very helpful because I was in a lot of pain'. She preferred the traditional midwife as a cheaper, more skilled alternative.

Views of obstetricians

For the two obstetricians (Dr One and Dr Two) I interviewed at Pt Villa hospital, the body was the primary risk because 'birth is a dangerous business' and because most women lived in poor, remote communities. Distance meant that surgery and caesarean sections to manage for high-risk birth – twins, breech, placenta praevia and post-partum haemorrhage – was not an option. As Dr One said, 'a baby after a CS [caesarean section] is more dangerous so we deliver them vaginally'. For Dr Two, the inherent risk in women's bodies was exacerbated by social determinants – lack of reliable transport in the event of post-partum haemorrhage and difficult labours (breech births, twins and obstructed delivery). In addition, traditional attendants who routinely used the kastom leaf compounded physiological risks of birth because:

> The kastom leaf intensifies the contractions, speeds up the labour and compromises the blood flow to the baby. Then the baby gets born flat and the traditional midwife cannot resuscitate the baby.

For Dr Two, traditional birth attendants ... 'were quite competent'. In contrast to Dr One, however, his approach was to formally incorporate them into the system training them to recognise emergencies (as is the maternity policy in Samoa). It was only when they were outside of the formal maternity system, unregulated and unregistered, that he felt that traditional attendants became a risk to women. Dr One, as the senior obstetrician, summarily dismissed the idea of incorporating traditional attendants not because they lacked skills but because of their cultural authority over younger women as:

> young women would think it was safe to birth in the village and whole referral system will collapse.

In Australia (where Dr One had worked for several years), he noted that the female body, ironically, represented a much higher risk than in Vanuatu because Australian women had fewer children, better education and nutrition and started families in their 30s (a medical risk factor for infertility):

> ... so infertility was higher. And when infertility is higher so the obstetrician is loathe to do anything wrong and women are told that CS [caesarean section] is the saviour; that it will not damage their pelvic muscles.

Caesarean section rates of over 35% were commonplace in Australia not due to risk health factors but due to cultural and social considerations such as 'practitioner convenience, patients' requests and high medical/legal costs'. As he explained, women's bodies were weaker too because those with a poorly structured pelvis who should have died had survived with better access to medical care, thus weakening the evolutionary chain. In Vanuatu, by contrast, women in remote villages whose forebears had survived were in better physiological shape to withstand the rigours of birth without an obstetrician although as they gravitated to the urban centres they too would become evolutionarily weaker. Dr One predicted that in the future Vanuatu women's bodies will pose grave risks to obstetricians, just as they do now in Western countries where many more women with poor pelvic structure necessitated high rates of surgical and other intervention and where obstetricians had lost the skills to deliver high-risk breech babies and twins. He noted that ni-Vanuatu obstetricians retained the skills to deliver difficult births (breech and twins) and were therefore highly valued in Western hospitals, but he was admonished for not performing more caesarean sections. As he explained, in Australia:

> every patient was a potential legal case whereas in Vanuatu we are short of blood, staff and resources and I work 24/7. If things go wrong [in Vanuatu] they will say it is an unfortunate situation.

He explained that he did his best and that in Vanuatu women were culturally attended to labour and none asked for morphine.

In short, although born in a developing country, Western training had given this obstetrician a typically Western approach to birth; he viewed bodies in general as fallible but female bodies were doubly dangerous. Physiologically and in evolutionary terms they were the primary site of risk for the baby and in cultural terms they were the primary site of risk for litigation – and thus for obstetricians' professional well-being.

Views of midwives

Midwives agreed with obstetricians that most of the risk of birthing in Vanuatu lay in the use of the kastom leaf, although there was no consensus on how this risk should be addressed. For senior staff like Jackie at Lenakel Hospital on Tanna Island:

kastom medicine is too strong for the baby and the heart beat is very high and some of them die. They get a bottle of kastom medicine and they hide it from us.

For Annette, senior midwife, at Nambawan Maternity Unit Blong Pt Villa Central Hospital, traditional practices were difficult to challenge:

...we cannot change that ... we cannot do anything with them, we cannot change their beliefs and we have to work with them. We respect their traditional ways, we have to work with them. We explain the risks of the kastom medicine, that it kills the mama and the baby.

Midwife Lisa located risk in the ignorance of the local elders in urging the young women to take the kastom leaf to accelerate contractions and make the labour quicker and easier because that was dangerous for the baby. For the same reason, Julie argued against the distribution of sterile birth packs because in their ignorance women would reuse them.

In relation to traditional birth attendants, some midwives were concerned about their lack of formal education in managing emergency obstetric conditions such as post-partum hae-morrhage and placenta praevia citing this as a high-risk factor in birth. Yet other midwives welcomed them in remote areas where women with high fertility rates (more than four pregnancies is deemed a medical risk factor) lacked access to trained health workers. For these midwives, traditional birth attendants could be used if only as an interim solution until more midwives were trained. (Although this would make it a long-term solution due to a small pool of post-secondary educated graduates.) Some midwives associated traditional attendants with high-risk factors due to their unhygienic practices and low levels of immunisation. Others, such as Betty (an antenatal registered nurse working at the health centre at Mele 20 minutes from Pt Villa), regarded social determinants, namely low income and poor transport, as contributing more to risk of child birth than traditional attendants and consider-ably traditional birth attendants could contribute to safe birth if they were trained and

have come to have some knowledge of training in washing hands before birth, how to cut the umbilical cord and how to sterilise things.

Others, like Lynda (the oldest midwife at Pt Vila hospital) and Julie, acknowledged the value of traditional attendants because they dealt with minor risks and practised safely and hygienically:

Yes, we trust them [traditional birth attendants]. We trained them in basic things like washing their hands, cleanliness and hygiene. I was born at home with one of those; they are very helpful. They make sure the women do not go through aggressive labour and the baby will be OK. So they are responsible nurses like us.

Sarah (the antenatal midwife at Pt Vila hospital) focused on social determinants – high fertility and compressed spacing – as the major risk factors noting that '...the women who have many births quickly, one year after another...' She argued that the birth itself and women's bodies were not major sites of risk because

it is natural for all women to give birth naturally and they need attend hospital or clinic only in the unlikely event that something went wrong.

For Ellen, the senior midwife, at Lenakel Hospital on Tanna, traditional attendants were not risky and neither were the so-called high-risk twin or breech births because they were routinely managed by midwives. She suggested that traditional attendants facilitated comprehensive coverage of women in villages. They could then have their first, fourth and subsequent births in hospital but stay with the traditional attendant in the village for the second and third births. Usually, she said, the traditional midwife in the village 'is very good and very skilled' and provided first advice to the young women after which they visited the nurse at the clinic (dispensary). For Julie, therefore, it was advisable to retain traditional attendants who were trained in hygiene and possessed demonstrable delivery skills because

> it was better to have someone in the village than no-one. They have been there for a long time, they are part of our culture … they are the people who are there all the time.

Views of traditional birth attendants

Although Leena was an urban-based birth attendant, her views were much like those of the other … traditional attendants I interviewed on remote Tanna. They saw risk as located, not in women's bodies or in birth or in following traditional practices such as using the kastom leaf to expedite labour, but in the domestic pressures on women that Leena said: '…caused them to do too much'. Leena and her mother had attended over 2000 births over the past 50 years and none of the women they had attended had died. They believed when pregnant women had had adequate rest and good nutrition, leafy greens, coconut milk, fish, chicken and pig meat and risks only increased when women were unable to eat the fresh and healthy island diet.

For Leena, the best and safest way for women to give birth was to stay in their village where the traditional birth attendant could use the kastom leaf to reduce the pain and speed up labour. She felt that staying at home was perfectly safe; her mother had taught her to manipulate a breech birth and administer bush herbs to stem any post-partum bleeding. As she pointed out, the health workers at the Pt Vila dispensary sought her assistance when mothers presented with high-risk conditions such as shoulder dystocia (although she was never formally paid). The biggest risk to mothers, she believed, was the loss of traditional midwifery tacit skills and knowledge since none of the young women in the village had any ambition to learn the old ways.

Discussion

From a largely dispersed, village-centred population living in over 65 islands where most inhabitants resided far from a clinic, hospital or health-aid post and where remote women must walk to the hospital in labour, women's decisions around the management of risk balanced the relative safety of birthplace, carer and ability to pay hospital fees and transport costs. No one option prevailed as the norm. All women navigated between traditional cosmological beliefs and practices and Western medical protocols. Despite negative sanction by obstetricians and midwives regarding use of the kastom leaf, women exercised cultural autonomy over use of bush medicines, over the use of traditional birth attendants, or not, or opting for the health post, clinic or hospital if traditional attendants were unavailable, unknown or untrusted. By contrast, the medical model of birth located risk primarily in women's bodies. For obstetricians and for many medically trained midwives, risk was also located in traditional beliefs and customs and especially in the cultural authority of pre-modern healers and birth attendants.

As a result, there are two parallel systems: traditional practices and bush medicines flourish alongside medical regimes and institutionalised birth. This was a hybridised culture of birth where risk was located in various objects and practices. Ni-Vanuatu women bridge the gap between Western and pre-modern practices by investing in elements of both paradigms to varying degrees according to their levels of trust and experience with traditional birth attendants, access to bush medicines, knowledge of hospital midwives and Western biomedicine, as well as their ability to pay for medical services and degree of proximity to hospitals and clinics. The only consistent marker among women seeking a 'good birth' – and thus their management of uncertainties including health and labour pain – was a universal trust in bush medicines. Communities harvested medicines for all kinds of maladies, but when women were in labour they used kastom leaf, against strong medical advice, to expedite labour and manage the acute pain of contractions. They were careful not to divulge this to medical practitioners and midwives to avoid being criticised as bad mothers. Traditional birth attendants were another point of contention. Some midwives could see the virtue of traditional attendants. Others did not. Obstetricians were divided; they strongly criticised the use of the kastom leaf, but some appreciated the tacit knowledge and skills of the traditional attendants. Yet this was not enough to expunge their fears that official endorsement and/or inclusion would dilute their own scientific authority and the hierarchical system of referral. In direct contrast to medical knowledge, traditional attendants remained confident in the ability of women to birth their babies. For them the real dangers were social; specifically, the normative assumption of women's onerous domestic responsibilities.

Given the complexities of this evidence – the diversity of interpretation and location of risks in childbirth among diverse social actors – it may be more accurate to think about risk in terms of risk *cultures* – groups that collectively endorse certain values and perceptions and who through cultural practices create unities and boundaries between themselves and Others. Use of the kastom leaf, for example, was deeply embedded in local cultures and could be seen as the hallmark of a hybridised culture where traditional medicines were widely used despite being contraindicated by medical knowledge; a fact known to women who continued to use it and to hide the fact from doctors and midwives (Douglas, 2002; Lash, 2000; Malinowksi, 1922). However, any unities were fluid and porous. Women's decisions about where to birth were not always driven by technical and scientific measurements of risk but by a range of contextual factors weighted in various ways. Obstetricians strenuously denied the utility of traditional attendants yet admired their skills. Exclusion meant defending Western medical authority which they knew was marginal, at best, in the face of the cultural authority of traditional healers and cosmologies. Midwives also regarded the use of the kastom leaf as a risky practice but knew that women would continue to use it. Most admired traditional birth attendants; some thought they should be incorporated into the system.

Conclusion

Attempts by governments in developing economies to centralise maternity care within a Westernised medical model have been only partially successful in Vanuatu. In traditional societies, like Vanuatu, where the biomedical model and Western cosmologies such as Christianity compete with pre-modern natural pharmacopoeia, such as the kastom leaf and traditional cosmologies, such as animism, women juggle various elements of both, depending upon individual circumstances. Traditional practices were widely embraced, and although many mothers accepted the idea of hospital as the safest location, they attended only briefly, while substantial advice in the prenatal and postnatal periods was sought from traditional attendants, if available. Or, put another way, the lens through which risk is viewed by the interpreter are multiplied so that the biomedical lens of risk is relativised. It carries authority but not absolute authority. A constructionist model of risk is thus much more appropriate because the evidence indicates that different actors find risk in different sites depending on their own social location and capacities and will gravitate towards practices, discourses and individuals they can trust, especially those with whom they feel a strong sense of community. Strategies are, therefore, formed less through scientific rationality but according to feelings and emotions and the lived experience. The concept of risk cultures conveys this complexity; they are formed around *values* rather than calculable rationalities. Risk cultures form self-reflexively to manage contingent circumstances.

A conventional positivist definition of risk where there is a consensus about site(s) of risk that may be forensically known in advance was not evident in the data I have used in this article. The implications for health policy in developing regimes are important. Medical knowledge may well benefit citizens, but planners would be advised to factor in local cultural mores and traditional practices when designing efficacious healthcare options.

Disclosure statement

No potential conflict of interest was reported by the author.

References

Abbott, A. (1988). *The system of the professions*. London: University of Chicago Press.

Alaszewski, A. (2003). Risk, trust and health. *Health, Risk & Society, 5*(3), 235–239. doi:10.1080/13698570310001606941

Alaszewski, A. (2015). Anthropology and risk: Insights into uncertainty, danger and blame from other cultures. *Health, Risk & Society, 17*(3/4). doi:10.1080/13698575.2015.1070128

Alaszewski, A. (in press). Risk, medicine and health. In A. Burgess & J. Zinn (Ed.), *Handbook of risk studies*. London: Routledge.

Alaszewski, A., & Burgess, A. (2007). Risk, time and reason. *Health, Risk & Society, 9*(4), 349–358. doi:10.1080/13698570701612295

Allen, D. (2002). Doing occupational demarcation: The boundary work of nurse managers in a district general hospital. In A. M. Rafferty & M. Traynor (Eds.), *Exemplary research for nursing and midwifery*. London: Routledge.

Ashford, L. (2014). *Hidden suffering: Disabilities from pregnancy and childbirth in less developed countries*. Washington, DC: Population Reference Bureau Measure Communication. Retrieved August 21, 2014, from http://www.prb.org/pdf/HiddenSufferingEng.pdf

Asian-Pacific Resource and Research Centre for Women (ARROW). (2001). *Redefining rights: Thematic studies series 4: Maternal mortality and morbidity in Asia* (Vol. 2011, p. 33). Kuala Lumpur: ARROW.

Barclay, L. (1997). Midwifery in Australia and surrounding regions. *Midwifery, 13*, 111–114. doi:10.1016/S0266-6138(97)90004-0

Beck, U. (1992). *Risk society: Towards a new modernity*. London: Sage.

Beck, U. (2009). *World risk society*. Malden, MA: Polity Press.

Bhutta, Z. A., Chopra, M., Axelson, H., Berman, P., Boerma, T., Bryce, J., ... Wardlaw, T. (2010). Countdown to 2015 decade report (2000–10): Taking stock of maternal, newborn, and child survival. *The Lancet, 375*, 2032–2044. doi:10.1016/S0140-6736(10)60678-2

Bowser, D., & Hill, K. (2010). *Exploring evidence for disrespect and abuse in facility-based childbirth*. Report of a Landscape Analysis for USAID-TRAction Project. Bethesda, MD: USAID, Harvard School of Public Health, University Research Co. LLC.

Bryers, H., & van Teijlingen, E. (2010). Risk, theory, social and medical models: A critical analysis of the concept of risk in maternity care. *Midwifery*, 26(5), 488–496. doi:10.1016/j.midw.2010.07.003

Byrne, A., & Morgan, A. (2011). How the integration of traditional birth attendants with formal health systems can increase skilled birth attendance. *International Journal of Gynecology & Obstetrics*, 115, 127–134. doi:10.1016/j.ijgo.2011.06.019

Chadwick, R. J., & Foster, D. (2014). Negotiating risky bodies: Childbirth and constructions of risk. *Health, Risk & Society*, 16(1), 68–83. doi:10.1080/13698575.2013.863852

Cheyne, H., Skar, S. S., Peterson, A., David, S., & Hodgkiss, F. (2013). *Having a baby in Scotland 2013: Women's experiences of maternity care. Volume 1: National results*. Stirling: Nursing, Midwifery and Allied Health Professions Research Unit, NHS, Scottish Government.

Coxon, K., Sandall, J., & Fulop, N. J. (2014). To what extent are women free to choose where to give birth? How discourses of risk, blame and responsibility influence birth place decisions. *Health, Risk & Society*, 16(1), 51–67. doi:10.1080/13698575.2013.859231

Coxon, K., Scamell, M., & Alaszewski, A. (2012). Risk, pregnancy and childbirth: What do we currently know and what do we need to know? An editorial. *Health, Risk & Society*, 14(6), 503–510. doi:10.1080/13698575.2012.709486

Creanga, A. A., Berg, C. J., Syverson, C., Seed, K. B. S., Bruce, F. C., & Callaghan, W. (2015). Pregnancy-related mortality in the United States, 2006–2010. *Obstetrics & Gynecology*, 125, 5–12. doi:10.1097/AOG.0000000000000564

Crook, S. (1999). Ordering risks. In D. Lupton (Ed.), *Risk and sociocultural theory* (pp. 160–185). Cambridge: Cambridge University Press.

De Vries, R., Benoit, C., van Teijlingen, E., & Wrede, S. (Eds.). (2001). *Birth by design: Pregnancy, maternity care and midwifery in North America and Europe*. London: Routledge.

Dean, M. (1999). Risk, calculable and incalculable. In D. Lupton (Ed.), *Risk and sociocultural theory* (pp. 131–159). Cambridge: Cambridge University Press.

Declercq, E., & Chalmers, B. (2008). Mothers' reports of their maternity experiences in the USA and Canada. *Journal of Reproductive and Infant Psychology*, 26(4), 295–308. doi:10.1080/02646830802408407

Dibben, M. R., & Lean, M. (2003). Achieving compliance in chronic illness management: Illustrations of trust relationships between physicians and nutrition clinic patients. *Health, Risk & Society*, 5(3), 241–258. doi:10.1080/13698570310001606950

Douglas, M. (1992). *Risk and blame: Essays in cultural theory*. London: Routledge.

Douglas, M. (2002). *Purity and danger: An analysis of concept of pollution and taboo*. Routledge Classic Edition. London: Routledge.

Douglas, M., & Wildavsky, A. (1982). *Risk and culture: An essay on the selection of technological and environmental dangers*. Berkeley, CA: University of California Press.

Ensor, T., & Cooper, S. (2004). Overcoming barriers to health service access: Influencing the demand side. *Health Policy and Planning*, 19, 69–79. doi:10.1093/heapol/czh009

Foucault, M. (1975). *The birth of the clinic: An archeology of medical perception*. New York, NY: Vintage Books.

Foucault, M. (1991). Governmentality. In G. Burchell, C. Gordon, & P. Miller (Eds.), *The Foucault effect: Studies in governmentality*. Hemel Hempstead: Harvester Wheatsheaf.

Fournier, V. (2000). Boundary work and the unmaking of the professions. In N. Malin (Ed.), *Professionalism, boundaries and the workplace*. London: Routledge.

Graham, W., Bell, J. S., & Bullough, H. W. (2001). Can skilled attendance at delivery reduce maternal mortality in developing countries? In V. De Brouwere & W. Van Lerberghe (Eds.), *Safe motherhood strategies: A recent review of the evidence*. Antwerp: ITGP Press.

Green, J. (1999). From accidents to risk: Public health and preventable injury. *Health, Risk & Society*, 1, 25–39. doi:10.1080/13698579908407005

Grosz, E. (1994). *Volatile bodies: Towards a corporeal feminism*. Bloomington: Indiana University Press.

Hacking, I. (1990). *The taming of chance*. Cambridge: Cambridge University Press.

Hallgrimsdottir, H. K., & Benner, B. E. (2014). 'Knowledge is power': Risk and the moral responsibilities of the expectant mother at the turn of the twentieth century. *Health, Risk & Society*, 16(1), 7–21. doi:10.1080/13698575.2013.866216

Henwood, K., Pidgeon, N., Sarre, S., Simmons, P., & Smith, N. (2008). Risk, framing and everyday life: Epistemological and methodological reflections from three socio-cultural projects. *Health, Risk & Society, 10*(5), 421–438. doi:10.1080/13698570802381451

Heyman, B., Alaszewski, A., & Brown, P. (2012). Health care through the 'lens of risk' and the categorisation of health risks – An editorial. *Health, Risk & Society, 14*(2), 107–115. doi:10.1080/13698575.2012.663073

Hoj, L., Da Silva, D., Hedegaard, K., Sandstrom, A., & Aaby, P. (2003). Maternal mortality: Only 42 days? *BJOG: An International Journal of Obstetrics and Gynaecology, 110*, 995–1000. doi:10.1016/S1470-0328(03)03907-7

Hunt, A. (2003). Risk and moralization in everyday life. In R. V. Ericson & A. Doyle (Eds.), *Risk and morality*. Toronto: University of Toronto Press.

Hurt, L. S., & Ronsmans, C. (2002). *Time since pregnancy and mortality in women of reproductive age in Matlab, Bangladesh*. Paper presented at the British Society for Population Studies, London, UK.

Katz-Rothman, B. (1996). Women, providers and control. *Journal of Obstetric, Gynaecologic & Neonatal Nursing, 25*(3), 253–256. doi:10.1111/j.1552-6909.1996.tb02433.x

Kruske, S., & Barclay, L. (2004). Effect of shifting policies on traditional birth attendant training. *Journal of Midwifery & Women's Health, 49*(4), 306–311. doi:10.1016/j.jmwh.2004.01.005

Lane, K. (1995). The medical model of the body as a site of risk: A case study of childbirth. In J. Gabe (Ed.), *Medicine, health and risk: Sociological approaches, sociology of' health and illness monograph series*. Oxford: Blackwell.

Lane, K. (2006). The plasticity of professional boundaries: A case study of collaborative care in maternity services. *Health Sociology Review, 15*(4), 341–352. doi:10.5172/hesr.2006.15.4.341

Lane, K. (2012). Dreaming the impossible dream: Ordering risks in Australian maternity care policies. *Health Sociology Review, 21*(1), 23–35. doi:10.5172/hesr.2012.21.1.23

Lane, K. L. (2013). *Health cosmopolitanism: The case for traditional birth attendants*. Melbourne: Centre for Citizenship and Globalisation. Research Paper Series. 4:1. May.

Lash, S. (2000). Risk culture. In B. Adam, U. Beck, & J. Van Loon (Eds.), *The risk society and beyond: Critical issues for social theory* (pp. 47–62). London: Sage.

Lash, S., Giddens, A., & Beck, U. (1994). *Reflexive modernization: Politics, tradition and aesthetics in the modern social order*. Cambridge: Polity Press.

Lassi, Z. S., Haider, B. A., & Bhutta, Z. A. (2010). Community-based intervention packages for reducing maternal and neonatal morbidity and mortality and improving neonatal outcomes. *Editorial Group, Cochrane Pregnancy and Childbirth Group*. Advance online publication. doi:10.1002/14651858.CD007754.pub2

Lothian, J. A. (2012). Risk, safety, and choice in childbirth. *The Journal of Perinatal Education, 21*(1), 45–47. doi:10.1891/1058-1243.21.1.45

Lupton, D. (1999). Introduction: Risk and sociocultural theory. In D. Lupton (Ed.), *Risk and sociocultural theory* (pp. 1–11). Cambridge: Cambridge University Press.

Lupton, D. (2013a). Risk and emotion: Towards an alternative theoretical perspective. *Health, Risk & Society, 15*(8), 634–647. doi:10.1080/13698575.2013.848847

Lupton, D. (2013b). *Risk* (2nd ed.). London: Routledge.

Malinowksi, B. (1922). *Argonauts of the Western Pacific*. London: Routledge.

Murphy-Lawless, J. (1998). *Reading birth and death: A history of obstetric thinking*. Bloomington: Indiana University Press.

Murray, C. J. L., & Lopez, A. D. (1998). Health dimensions of sex and reproduction. In *Global burden of disease and injury series* (p. 3). Boston, MA: Harvard University Press.

Ostlin, P., Eckermann, E., Mishra, U. S., Nkowane, M., & Wallstam, E. (2006). Gender and health promotion: A multisectoral policy approach. *Health Promotion International, 21*(Supplement 1), 25–35. doi:10.1093/heapro/dal048

Peace Corps Vanuatu. (2013). Retrieved May 18, 2013, from http://vanuatu.peacecorps.gov/content/history-culture

Pickstone, J., & Cooter, R. (2000). *Medicine in the twentieth century*. Singapore: Harwood Academic Publishers.

Power, M. (1997). *The audit society: Rituals of verification*. Oxford: Oxford University Press.

Quandl. (2013). Retrieved from http://www.quandl.com/society/vanuatu-all-society-indicators

RANZCOG. (2011). Homebirth. *RANZCOG Magazine, 13*(4).

Ray, A. M., & Salihu, H. M. (2004). The impact of maternal mortality interventions using traditional birth attendants and village midwives. *Journal of Obstetrics & Gynaecology, 24*(1), 5–11. doi:10.1080/01443610310001620206

Reisman, C. K. (1983). Women and medicalization: A new perspective. *Social Policy, 14*(1), 3–18.

Ronsmans, C., & Graham, W. J. (2006). The Lancet Maternal Survival Series steering group. Maternal mortality: Who, when, where, and why. *The Lancet, 368*, 1189–1200. doi:10.1016/S0140-6736(06)69380-X

Rothfield, P. (1995). Bodies and subjects: Medical ethics and feminism. In P. Komesaroff (Ed.), *Troubled bodies: Critical perspectives on postmodernism, medical ethics and the body*. London: Duke University Press.

Rothman, B. K. (2014). Pregnancy, birth and risk: An introduction. *Health, Risk & Society, 16*(1), 1–6. doi:10.1080/13698575.2013.876191

Scamell, M., & Alaszewski, A. (2012). Fateful moments and the categorisation of risk: Midwifery practice and the ever-narrowing window of normality during childbirth. *Health, Risk & Society, 14*(2), 207–221. doi:10.1080/13698575.2012.661041

Shilling, C. (2003). *The body and social theory* (2nd ed.). London: Sage.

Sibley, L., Sipe, T. A., & Koblinsky, M. (2004). Does traditional birth attendant training improve referral of women with obstetric complications: A review of the evidence. *Social Science & Medicine, 59*, 1757–1768. doi:10.1016/j.socscimed.2004.02.009

Starrs, A. (1997). *The safe motherhood action agenda: Priorities for the next decade*. New York, NY: Inter-agency Group for Safe Motherhood and Family Care International.

The Royal Society. (1992). *Risk: Analysis, perception and management. Report of a Royal Society study group*. London: The Royal Society.

Tonkiss, F. (2006). *Contemporary economic sociology: Globalisation, production, inequality*. London: Routledge.

Tulloch, J., & Lupton, D. (2003). *Risk and everyday life*. London: Sage.

Turner, B. S. (2014). Risks, rights and regulation: An overview. *Health, Risk & Society, 3*(1), 9–18.

Wagner, M. (1994). *Pursuing the birth machine: The search for appropriate birth technology*. Sevenoaks, Kent: ACE Graphics.

Wagner, M. (2001). Fish can't see water: The need to humanize birth. *International Journal of Gynecology & Obstetrics, 75*(1), S25–S37. doi:10.1016/S0020-7292(01)00519-7

Walraven, G., & Weeks, A. (1999). The role of (traditional) birth attendants with midwifery skills in the reduction of maternal mortality. *Tropical Medicine and International Health, 4*(8), 527–529. doi:10.1046/j.1365-3156.1999.00441.x

Walsh, D. (2007). *Evidence-based care for normal labour & birth: A guide for midwives*. London: Routledge.

Walsh, D., & Downe, S. (2004). Outcomes of free-standing, midwidery-led birth centres: A structured review of the evidence. *Birth, 31*(3), 222–229. doi:10.1111/bir.2004.31.issue-3

World Bank. (2013). Retrieved September 3, 2013, from wits.worldbank.org/Country Profile/VUT

World Health Organisation. (1997). *The world health report 1997 conquering suffering enriching humanity*. Geneva: Author.

World Health Organization. (1992). *Traditional birth attendants: A joint WHO/UNICEF/UNFPA statement*. Geneva: Author.

World Health Organization. (1996). *Essential newborn care: Report of a technical working group*. WHO/FRH/MSM/96. Geneva: Author.

World Health Organization. (2014). *World health statistics*. Geneva: Author. Retrieved May, 2014, from http://apps.who.int/iris/bitstream/10665/112738/1/9789240692671_eng.pdf

Zinn, J. (2008). Introduction: The contribution of sociology to the discourse on risk and uncertainty. In J. Zinn (Ed.), *Social theories of risk and uncertainty* (pp. 1–17). Oxford: Blackwell.

Time, risk and midwife practice: the vaginal examination

Mandie Scamell[a] and Mary Stewart[b]

[a]School of Health Sciences, City University, London, UK; [b]MRC Centre of Epidemiology for Child Health, UCL Institute of Child Health, University College London, London, UK

In this article, we examine the impact on midwifery practice of clinical governance in the UK with its shift from individual autonomous practice based on personal experience and intuition (embodied knowledge) to the collective control of work based on guidelines and protocols (encoded knowledge) associated with the scientific–bureaucratic approach to care. We focus on the ways in which midwives use partograms and associated vaginal examinations to monitor and manage the progress of labour. The partogram represents (among other things) a timetable for dilation of the cervix during labour. Women who fail to keep up with this timetable are shifted from a low-to-high risk category and subjected to additional surveillance and intervention. In this article, we draw on empirical evidence taken from two independent ethnographic studies of midwifery talk and practice in England undertaken in 2005–2007 and 2008–2010, to describe the ways in which midwives practice of vaginal examinations during labour both complies with, while at the same time creatively subverts, the scientific–bureaucratic approach to maternity care. We argue that although divergent in nature, each way of practicing is mutually dependent upon the other: the space afforded by midwifery creativity not only co-exists with the scientific–bureaucratic approach to care, but also sustains it.

Introduction

In this article, we examine the impact on professional practice of clinical governance, measures designed to standardise professional decision-making using clinical evidence to reduce risks and increase efficiency. We examine the ways in which midwives are expected to manage labour and childbirth undertaking regular and intimate vaginal examination of mothers in labour to ensure that their labour is safe and 'on time'. When midwife examinations indicate that the labour is too slow and does not conform to the anticipated timetable then it becomes high risk and subject to medical intervention. It is not our intention in the article to dispute the pervasiveness of the evidence-based approach to midwifery care which underpins practice, nor do we mean to challenge the enormity of its hold upon the midwifery imagination, the data that we use in this article and other data that we have published elsewhere (Scamell 2011, Scamell and Alaszewski 2012) provide adequate evidence for what Brown and Crawford (2003) aptly refer to as the self-regulation of 'deep management' where practitioners police themselves to ensure practice is standardised. What we aim to do in this article is to use ethnographic evidence to engage with the ways midwives make sense of the limitations set out by the risk management mechanisms of clinical governance and how they creatively find space for both personal and professional autonomy.

We start this article with a background section that provides a brief introductory overview of current midwifery activity in the National Health Service (NHS) and the technology of risk as it operates within the NHS maternity care provision in the UK. We then move on to discuss the research studies that provided the data which we use in this article. In the main findings section of the article, we use data from our field notes and interviews to examine how risk crystallises into meaningful action through midwifery talk and practice. We examine how institutional, clinical governance concerns with risk can underpin organisational technologies which centre on the standardisation of care and the timing of that care through the strict adherence to institutional protocols and meticulous record keeping. Yet at the same time, more covert meaning-making activities around risk exist. In the discussion section, we develop the principle proposition that the success of the maternity service provision operates upon diverse and concurrent ways of knowing about and working with risk.

Controlling professional practice: clinical governance, midwifery practice and the management of labour

Clinical governance and the standardisation of midwifery care

When the NHS was created in the UK in the 1940s, individual clinicians in the new service were granted clinical autonomy, the right to manage and regulate their own work. However since the 1980s, successive governments have seen such individual autonomy as problematic, creating both costs and risks which have been evident in inquiries into avoidable harm and death (Alaszewski 2003, Alaszewski and Brown 2012, pp. 114–139).

In 1997, the response of the new Labour Government was to launch a new initiative to improve the quality of professional practice and reduce risk through clinical governance which was defined as:

> A new initiative … to assure and improve clinical standards at the local level throughout the NHS. This includes action to ensure that risks are avoided, adverse events are rapidly detected, openly investigated and lessons learned, good practice is rapidly disseminated and systems are in place to ensure continuous improvements in clinical care. (DH 1997)

Clinical governance involves a major shift in the management of professional practice from a system based on individual autonomy in which individual practitioners base their decisions and practice on their professional judgement developed through personal knowledge and experience to a system based on collective self-regulation in which all professional decisions are grounded in encoded knowledge (Lam 2000) and are evidence-based, so that there is a systematic and uniform approach to decision-making and practice. As Flynn (2000) notes that there is a tension in modern society 'between decisions governed by formalised rules and procedures, and action determined by tacit knowledge and individual expertise'. Clinical governance seeks to resolve this tension through the use of formalised rules and procedures. Clinical governance is a form of collective self-regulation based on what Harrison refers to as *scientific–bureaucratic* medicine with standardised timetables (Harrison and Wood 2000, p. 26).

Clinical governance and midwifery: timetables and vaginal examinations

The National Institute for Health and Clinical Excellence (2007), a government-funded 'arms-length' agency, has established guidelines for maternity practice. These guidelines specify that all settings in which women give birth should come under the 'oversight ... of multidisciplinary clinical governance structures (p. 10)' and that all individual births should be subject to surveillance and checking:

> In all places of birth, risk assessment in the antenatal period and when labour commences should be subject to continuous audit. (The National Institute for Health and Clinical Excellence 2007, p. 10)

The National Institute for Health and Clinical Excellence guidelines (2007, p. 33) provides a framework for the midwife decision-making and activity by dividing normal labour into three stages based on timed physiological activities. Childbirth is carved up into delineated stages, each with its own timeframe parameter (see Table 1) and midwives are expected to diligently monitor the progress of the labour and to measure and record the dilation of the cervix on a graph or partogram which NICE describes as:

> A pictorial record of labour (partogram) should be used once labour is established ... Where the partogram includes an action line, the World Health Organization recommendation of a 4-hour action line should be used. (The National Institute for Health and Clinical Excellence 2007, p. 26)

The guidelines indicate that midwives should monitor the progress of labour through an intimate and intrusive action, a vaginal examination. The guidelines indicate that following a vaginal examination that identifies the cervix is 4 cm dilated and labour is established, the midwife should ask to examine a woman every 4 hr (The National Institute for Health and Clinical Excellence 2007) to ensure that she does not experience increased risks by labouring for too long.

A vaginal examination is an intimate, internal clinical examination performed by midwives (and/or obstetricians) and the stated purpose of this examination is to assess

Table 1. NICE definition of stages and time limits.

Stages and sub-stages	Definition	Time limits
First stage of labour	From the onset of labour until full dilation of the cervix (10 cm)	First baby, average 8 hr, maximum 15 hr Subsequent, average 5 hr, maximum 12 hr
Established labour	Regular painful contraction during which cervix fully dilates from 4 to 10 cm	Cervix should dilate at least 2 cm in 4 hr Dilation should not slow
Second stage of labour Passive phase	Full cervical dilation in the absence of involuntary expulsion contractions	
Active phase	Baby visible and involuntary expulsion contractions and/or active mothers effort to give birth	First baby 3 hr, intervention after 2 hr Subsequent babies 2 hr, intervention after 1 hr
Third stage of labour	Following the birth of the baby, the expulsion of afterbirth and membranes	30 min with active management and 60 min with physiological

progress of the labour. The vaginal examination can be seen as being part of the safety technology employed by practitioners to reduce risk by ensuring and protecting the wellbeing of mother and child. The premises upon which the routine practice of vaginal examination rests are that:

- spontaneous labour follows a predictable and lineal timetable;
- labour progress can and should be measured against this expected timetable;
- progress should be both closely monitored and recorded in the maternal notes – using a partogram – and that midwives should intervene if a woman's labour lags too far behind the expected timetable;
- without this surveillance birth is more risky, with increased risk of harm to both the mother and baby.

Although the evidence base for this timetable is not clear and midwife researchers have expressed concerns about the routine use of the partogram to monitor all labours (Lavender et al. 2008, Schmid and Downe 2010, Walsh 2010), the performance of regular vaginal examinations in labour to assess both progress and risk continues to be a crucial component of standardised midwifery practice in the UK (Shepherd and Cheyne 2012). Both the authors of this article as practicing midwives in the UK have experienced the expectation to assess the progress of all labour using vaginal examinations, to check whether the labour is 'on-time', that is conforms to the partogram timetable (Groeschel and Glover 2001, Stewart 2005, Russell 2007, Scamell 2011). As the partogram creates a prescriptive health trajectory or timetable, once recognised and legitimised through routine activity, it becomes the duty of health-care professionals to detect any deviations from that norm (Armstrong 1995). Midwives practicing in the UK are responsible and accountable for ensuring that each individual labour is subject to constant surveillance through the practice of regular vaginal examinations in an effort to detect risk and normalise (through medical intervention) those labours which are deemed to be too slow and by implication therefore deviate from what is assumed to be low risk labour (Simonds 2002, Downe and Dykes 2009, Scamell 2011).

We have noted in this section that health care in the UK has shifted from a system of clinical autonomy with independent practitioners using their knowledge and experience to make decisions and manage risk to a system of clinical governance in which professional practice is collectively managed through a system of agreed rules and procedures creating a scientific–bureaucratic approach to care. Individual midwives are required to use an agreed timetable embodied in the partogram to manage labour so that they identify labours that are too slow and take action to minimise potential risk to mother and baby. To maintain their surveillance of the cervix, midwives are expected to undertake regular and intrusive internal vaginal examinations. The current empirical basis for showing how midwives undertake this work is limited, and the main debates centre largely on the ethics of informed consent for the procedure rather than its potential benefits or risks (e.g., see Bergstrom *et al.* 1992, Stewart 2004). In this article, we explore the interpretive work midwives have to do when translating the scientific–bureaucratic approach to care, set out through institutionalised protocol, procedure and record keeping, into meaningful action.

Methodology: two studies

In this article, we draw on data from two UK-based ethnographic research studies that used field study methods, participant observation and linked interviews in NHS birthing settings to examine the ways in which midwives organised and talked about their work. The two studies were both carried out by 'indigenous ethnographers', that is midwife practitioner researchers but they had distinct foci:

- Study I examined midwives' and women's experiences of vaginal examination in labour.
- Study II examined how midwives made sense of and talked about risk.

However given the centrality of partogram timetable and its links to vaginal examination, both studies provided rich data on how and in what ways individual midwives used partograms and how this shaped their practice, management of risk and interactions with birthing mothers, especially through vaginal examinations. As we will show in the findings section, there was an amount of consistency between the findings of the two studies, even though the two investigations were geographically and historically distinct in that they were separated by 3 years and around 300 miles.

Both the studies used to inform that this article had an interest in the micro-analysis of midwifery talk and practice. Although this research design was applied in broadly the same way, the emphasis and framing were slightly different in the two. Study I took place in the West of England and involved 20 women and 10 midwives and was based on a feminist critical ethnographic approach (Stacey 1988, Naples 2003). This investigation took place between 2005 and 2007 and the researcher concentrated on exploring midwives' and women's experiences of vaginal examination in labour. Study II adopted an ethnographic discourse analysis approach (Gwyn 2002) with an emphasis on sociolinguistics, examining not only practice but more particularly the ways in which midwives talked about and reflected on practice and in particular risk. This study took place between 2008 and 2010 in the South of England and the researcher worked alongside and talked to 33 midwives responsible for the delivery of intrapartum care in various clinical settings.

Both researchers were qualified midwives who engaged in participant observation, observing and talking to midwives about their practice and recording their observations and conversations in detailed ethnographic field notes and ethnographic interviews. In both studies, data analysis took place alongside data collection so that emerging findings influenced choices around data collection techniques, sampling target interview structure and so on. In Study II, analysis was aided by the qualitative data analysis software Atlas ti. In Study I, all analyses were performed manually.

Access and ethics

In Study I, the midwifery participants were accessed through the primary sample group of 20 birthing women. The researcher attended the labours of these women and thereby gained access to her secondary sample – the midwives. The second study took a very different approach to recruitment which involved self-selection following a recruitment and information campaign targeted at all midwives working in the selected sites; subsequent recruitment was achieved through opportunistic, snowball technique (Bryman 2004) with some attention to purposeful structuring to maximise diversity recruiting 33 midwives. Written consent and sequential verbal consent (Parker 2007) were gained from all those involved in both studies and all transcripts and field notes were 'cleaned', with identifying features removed, prior to analysis and all the names used in this article are pseudonyms. Both researchers obtained the required research governance approvals through the sponsoring organisations and the hosting NHS Trusts. The Heads of Risk,

Assurance and Legal Services and the Heads of Midwifery of the relevant services reviewed and approved the project protocols before the fieldwork started.

Findings

In this section of the article, we will examine the ways in which the midwives in our study responded to and managed the scientific–bureaucratic, institutional protocols designed to guide their practices and ensure that they identified and managed risk correctly. We are particularly interested in how and when these midwives felt that they had to breach these protocols in relation to the performance of and recording of the vaginal examination.

Self-regulation and the standardisation of care

All the 43 midwives involved in the two research projects were uneasy with the idea of rule breaking; they tended to see this as unnecessary risk taking. They perceived risks stemming from such activity ranging from risk to the mother and baby to risks to themselves as practitioners but regardless of the loci of risk, what was quite clear from our data was that the participants in our studies were unwilling to condone non-compliance to the standardisation of care that they saw as being grounded in the encoded knowledge that underpinned the institution's protocols and guidelines. Despite a constant interest in what was called 'normal birth' and the constraints imposed by a protocol driven, standardisation approach to maternity care, as Andrea, a senior community midwife involved in Study II, pointed out, encoded knowledge provided the context or 'boundary' for individual decisions:

> I understand the need for protocols and guidelines because otherwise you wouldn't know who was who and what was what. So I think you need those boundaries but within [these] I think you need to assess each individual on their own merit and make their particular plan based on the whole picture.

When asked about their adherence to the protocols, midwives in our studies were often keen to acknowledge their understanding of the requirements for adherence. Dianna, for example, another community based midwife in Study II saw her practice bound by the institution's protocols aimed at standardising care:

> *Researcher*: So in some respects protocols can restrict your better judgement?
>
> *Dianna*: I think in some respects they are, they can. We are always told that protocols are there for guidelines they don't have to be abided by. Having said that, if you go against the protocols people are likely to haul you up on it. Every time. (Study II)

Hilary, a midwifery manager in Study II, said that she felt that her contract of employment made her feel obliged to adhere to protocols even when she did not agree with them:

> 'erm, just because, because I signed a contract with them that I feel duty bound to adhere to the variety of different protocols and guidelines that have been put in place for me to work by. I don't agree with a lot of them … I just think, I can't, I just have to go along with what they say even if I don't agree with it. (Study II)

What Hilary was describing was the multiplicity of meaning making where disparate ideas about the nature of birth and the nature of risk in birth interface. Hilary, like the majority of participants in both of these ethnographic studies, defended a position where childbirth could be imagined, even revered, as being a normal physiological event. At the same time however, Hilary felt that all midwives were obliged to acquiesce to the standardised care set out in the institutional guidelines, even when the activities associated with encoded knowledge were perceived as threatening this professional commitment to normal birth.

All the midwives recognised that the partogram timetable and the associated surveillance of labouring mothers were a key component of the protocols and guidelines that provided the framework for their decisions and practice. Debbie, a community midwife participating in Study I, when describing transferring birthing women from home to hospital talked about how the pressure to conform to prescriptive care protocols and in particular to undertake vaginal examinations so she could let staff know how dilated the cervix was. Debbie often felt compelled to do a vaginal examination so that provide the information required by the 'regular system':

> I have felt I needed to know what the cervix was doing before being able to transfer them in [to hospital] because I knew I'd be joining the regular system and they wouldn't tolerate me saying 'Oh I don't know how dilated she is'. (Study I)

Although the rationale for complying with the standardisation of care varied from an understanding of professional regulation, employee duty of care and tacit understandings of the interpersonal relations in the institutional setting, when we asked directly about protocols and guidelines all the midwives in our study stated that they were willing and able to work within the guideline and protocols. In other words, all the participants accepted the standardisation of care and practice as encoded in and represented by institutional guidelines, even when they felt that these protocols might not necessarily support good practice. They concurred with the importance of minimising risk in maternity care and accepted that compliance with set protocols was a way to minimise risk. Indeed, when protocol-based, standardised practice was explicitly challenged, the reaction of the midwives tended to be critical and hostile. For example in Study II, the researcher took part in a NHS staff study session in which an independent midwife described allowing a mother to labour 'in her own' time and therefore not following the NICE partogram timetable. During the discussion that followed the presentation, several of the midwives made little effort to hide their contempt openly saying 'that's just ridiculous. No it's worse than that, it's darn right dangerous.' When the independent midwife tried to defend her practice, another NHS midwife said: 'Well that may well be how you do it, dear, but it is not how we do things in the NHS. I would hate to be an independent midwife.' In this instance, the NHS midwives' commitment to encoded knowledge and NHS standardised care associated with this knowledge was sufficient to reframe midwifery commitment to normal birth as a site of risk. Practices associated with this risk were clearly regarded with contempt.

Other hidden ways of knowing: using intuition and experience

However, nestling quietly alongside this apparent acceptance of the organisation's clinical governance agenda and its commitment to minimising risk were other more covert and subversive ways of knowing and doing. This hidden knowledge was in many instances irreconcilable with the standardisation of care principal of clinical governance. This is not to say that these midwives were ever in the business of ignoring risk, on the contrary their hidden knowledge and covert activity centred around a concern to reduce risk. The reason this less visible way of being a midwife was at odds with the encoded knowledge ratified through the institution's risk management technologies was because it involved a process of risk reframing where tacit professional discretion and intuition could be legitimately expressed and acted upon. Interestingly those midwives, who openly talked about relying upon hidden knowledge in their daily work, understood that expressions of such tacit midwifery could only take place at the margins of daily activity. For example, Silvia, a senior midwife working in a birth centre described how she managed some labours, explaining that she just knew:

> That baby is just going to come. And that is intuition. We do use intuition but we know ... if someone sat in front of me, when a mistake has been made and I say: 'I used intuition', they are going to say: 'What are you talking about?' So that is the world we live in, isn't it? I suppose official midwifery can be quite different from actual midwifery? (Study II)

Here, Silvia was talking about her intuitive knowledge, a knowledge that is marginal and underpins the trust that the baby will come, that birth is a normal physiological process, a process that does not demand medical intervention or management.

Mary, a community midwife explained how this hidden knowledge worked:

> We are told with our notes ... you, you write your notes very carefully because basically for the next 25 years you can be called to account for them. And how can you possibly put in there, 'my instinct tells me that'? So it is one of those things that you have got to keep to yourself or maybe share, you know I will sometimes say, when you do a hand-over I will sometimes say 'Actually I haven't been very happy with this or that.' (Study II)

In contrast to Silvia, Mary's hidden knowledge was driven by a suspicion of pathology rather than a nebulous faith in normality. Intuitive midwifery knowledge operated in complex ways both confirming and unsettling professional commitments to understanding childbirth as a normal physiological event. What was clear from the evidence that we collected in both of the studies was that the midwives were aware of protocols with their encoded knowledge but they also recognised less visible and more personal ways of knowing, such as intuition.

Risk reframing: vaginal examinations and the partogram timetable

Given the strict timetable encoded in the partogram, midwives in both studies had developed practices that gave them a degree of control of and flexibility within the timetable. In Study II, Donna a community midwife referred to 'the midwife's VE' (vaginal examination) when describing the ways in which she and her colleagues did not accurately record their findings, for example delaying recording that the cervix had dilated to 4 cm, and therefore delaying the diagnosis of established labour:

> *Donna*: Well, you can always do a midwife's VE [vaginal examination] of course [laughs].
>
> *Researcher*: What is that?
>
> *Donna*: I'm not sure I should say [laughs]. Oh well, you know, it is a time when you have to be a bit ... you know, liberal with how you record your findings. (Study II)

Midwives were concerned that when they identified the onset of established labour, they were effectively starting a clock and this would lead to an implementation of a raft of seemingly benign intensive surveillance technologies to ensure the labour went to timetable and if it did there would be another set of interventions. Therefore, midwives could and did use creative acts of discretion to prevent the clock starting. For example, the following extract is from a conversation between a midwife, Jane, and a labouring woman, Samantha, following a vaginal examination that took place shortly after her admission. The examination indicated that Samantha was 5 cm dilated and therefore in established labour but as the following extract from field notes indicates Jane the midwife chose to record it as 2–3 cm there was 'no need' to start the more intensive surveillance:

> Jane told her (the mother) that she had done well but that she was in the early stages of her labour.

> 'Between you and me,' she said 'your cervix can stretch right up to five centimetres but we shan't write that down just yet, there is no need. It will only mean a load of hassle.'

> Jane recorded in the notes that the cervix was two to three centimetres dilated; importantly, Samantha (the mother) was not diagnosed as in labour …

> Later, during handover, Jane described Samantha as being five centimetres dilated, but explained to the midwives who were taking over care that she hadn't bothered putting it in the notes like that. None of the on-coming staff reacted negatively to this, they nodded in approval. (Field Notes Study II)

The reaction of the other midwives in the staffroom during this handover was particularly interesting as it suggested that the underestimating of examination results, in relation to cervical dilatation, was common practice. For example, Miranda an experienced midwife described how she systematically delayed recording the start of established labour:

> When they [labouring mothers] are 4 cm … and then in which case I will try to make them 3 and not 4 and then they are not in established labour. Well if I re-examined her (four hours later) if she is not in established labour … so she could be the same and so I could say to her 'Well actually, this is, you have not laboured. You are about the same so we can wait a bit longer for you to get into established labour'. (Study I)

This practice has been recorded elsewhere in the professional literature indicating that this may be accepted, albeit covert practice (Stewart 2004, Russell 2007). The rationale for this practice was to postpone the onset of intensive surveillance and was spoken about freely during midwife–midwife, and even midwife–client, talk. By underestimating Samantha's dilatation, Jane was able to avoid having to commence labour care monitoring, allowing Samantha to labour at her own, individual pace, which might or might not fall within the standardised protocol trajectory. Or put another way, by recasting the encoded knowledge underpinning the standardised management of labour protocol as a source of risk in itself, Jane, with the approval of the other oncoming midwifery staff, was able to privilege a professional judgement which functioned to subvert the confines set by the institution's rules.

Midwives indicated that they wanted to minimise risks to the pregnant women and at times saw the prescribed pathways and timetables as potentially hazardous. This meant that at crucial points in the process when the clock started ticking, start of established labour and onset of birth, midwives created 'grey areas' that enabled them to delay the start of the clock. As Nina an obstetric unit midwife noted how she delayed the 'end' of the first stage of labour when her experience and personal knowledge indicated that a woman needed more time for a normal birth by recording that there was an anterior lip, that is the baby's head had not quite passed out of the womb into the vagina:

I might document that there's an anterior lip[1] when there isn't and that … a lot of that is because I know I'm going to get a normal delivery in here but I know it's going to take [the woman] a bit longer and I don't want them to start pushing yet so if I say she's an anterior lip that'll buy us a bit more time. (Study II)

Participants from both studies felt that they had to use their own experience and considered professional judgement to 'make the system' work and to override the timetable or at least delay the start of the clock when they felt that the labouring woman could do with more opportunity to birth spontaneously. However, there were also occasions on which midwives created time by delaying the clock to suit their own convenience. For example, in Study I there was some evidence of self-interested manipulation of time. For example, Nina who indicated that she identified a 'lip' to buy a labouring women time also acknowledged that she sometimes invented a lip if she was coming to end of her shift and wanted to pass responsibility on a midwife on the next shift:

Conversely, if [the woman is] fully [dilated] and I'm going home in a minute, I don't want [her] to start pushing … I'm going to turn her on her side and say she's got a lip and let the next person take over. (Study I)

The midwives in both studies were willing to disregard the partogram timetable when they felt it was safe to do so and when there were potential benefits, usually for the labouring women but on occasion for themselves. However, data from Study I show that when midwives did disregard the official timetable they sometimes felt the need to reassure themselves that the labour was progressing satisfactorily and to do this some midwives adopted a covert strategy to gather more clinical information on the progress of the labour. They undertook undocumented vaginal examinations, sometimes without the permission of the labouring mothers. These covert examinations were referred to as: *the quickie*. An obstetric unit midwife, Gemma, described the quickie in the following way:

Gemma: Oh the quickie, well, a quickie, you have a quick feel to see what you're doing. yeah.

Researcher: And what's the difference between a quickie and a regular vaginal examination?

Gemma (without any hesitation): Oh the quickie's undocumented. (Study I)

For some midwives, the unofficial quickie has become part of routine practice. For example, in Study I, the researcher recorded the use of the quickie in the following way:

Anna (the mother) was in the second stage of labour and, although I could not see what was happening, I hear her give a small yelp of discomfort and protest 'Ow!'

Belinda, the midwife, apologised saying 'OK, just checking'. It was apparent that she had done a vaginal examination without consent and I am shocked at what I have just witnessed.

In some birthing units, the disregard of the official partogram timetable and the use of the quickie to monitor women's labour were part of routine albeit covert practice. Claire an experienced midwife from Study I described how she observed and learnt about covert examinations, in her terms 'dip ins', in the birthing unit she trained in:

Well, when I was in the unit where I trained I used to notice there were two ways in which the qualified midwives practised, and one was the big procedure and the four-hourly thing, and the other was they used to dip in all the time! We weren't encouraged to do that, it was sort of 'don't look at me, I'm just going to find something out'. (Study I)

Developing an alternative approach to practice: managing documents

Although midwives claimed that they accepted the principals of clinical governance, with its emphasis on standardised care grounded in official timetable to ensure safety and minimise risk, in practice they often subverted and disregarded the official timetable and engaged in covert forms of practice, for example, doing quickies. Effectively different ways of knowing about birth and being a midwife co-existed. The drivers behind this creativity were diverse, ranging from a concern to provide mothers with an opportunity for a normal birth to managing the conflicting demands of the job.

The disregard of the official partogram timetable and the use of alternative techniques to monitor the progress of labour such as the quickie were so systematic that they formed part of an alternative form of midwife practice, albeit one which was covert. For example, Claire an experienced midwife in her description of unsanctioned and undocumented vaginal examinations described them as a part of an unofficial practice contrasting them to the official way of doing things, 'the big procedure and the four-hourly thing'.

This approach was based on alternative source of knowledge, midwives accumulated expertise and experience that underpinned their professional discretion. Andrea, an experienced midwife, indicated that while she accepted the need for partogram timetable when she felt that labour was progressing albeit a bit slowly she was willing to use her judgement to give a labouring mother a bit more time:

> If I think 'Now this woman can do this on her own, just give her another half an hour everything is okay' so then you negotiate at the point I think rather than sweep everyone along with the guideline. (Study II)

A key element in this alternative approach to practice is the management of information and recording. As we have already noted some midwives deliberately under documented the findings from vaginal examinations so that they could retain professional discretion. As Karen, a hospital midwife, indicated that she concealed information that a woman was fully dilated and therefore ready to give birth by underreporting her finding and reducing the chance that there would be medical intervention that would curtail the length of labour:

> Oh (laughing) I was with a woman last week and I assessed her and she was fully [dilated] and I just thought 'They [the doctors] don't need to know that' so I wrote down that she was 8 cms [dilated]'. (Study I)

By under recording her findings in the medical records, Karen was able to actively by-pass the limitations imposed by policy-based surveillance regimes in an effort to create space where the mother could labour *in her own time*. Through this creativity, this midwife was able to reframe her risk priorities and express her professional discretion rather than confine her practice to the scientific–bureaucratic restraints set by the labour progress trajectory set down through the hospital's partogram and protocols. By under recording the mother's cervical dilatation in the official record, Karen bought herself and the labouring mother she was caring for some time. Midwives were willing to set aside the official timetable and clock to give mothers' time and space. They trusted the mother's body. As Susan a midwife in Study II put it:

But still the thrill the amazing thrill of the labour and the birth and what women do it never ceases to amaze me. You look at women and you listen to what they have to say and you think right you know she can do it. You know she will give birth beautifully you just need, she just needs time. We just need to give her the the the space to do it and she will.

The midwives in our studies used both adherence to risk technology and flouting it as a means of asserting their professional identity and autonomy. The restraints on practice posed by the scientific–bureaucratic approach to care, and the regimented timing of that care, were at once revered and actively subverted. In some instances, the midwives involved in these studies saw the risk technologies of the scientific–bureaucratic approach as a security, protecting the mother from the inherent risks of childbirth. At the same time, these technologies were seen to pose risks in themselves to the mothers in their care. This multiplicity of meaning making meant that the participants in these studies could shift effortlessly from positions of defence to covert resistance depending upon the nature of the professional identity they were defending through their talk and practice. For example, the mother's embodied birthing clock could be used as a justification for professional discretion and a way of resisting medical intervention as Karen described; if the doctors did not know that the woman she was caring for was fully dilated they could not intervene. Conversely, in a different context adherence and proof of rigid adherence to the timetable set out in the institutional protocols could be used to mark of professionalism as the data at the beginning of the findings section showed. Here, adherence to the institutional timetables was not only desirable, it provided practitioners with the moral high ground from which 'dangerous' and 'unprofessional' independent midwifery practice could be rejected.

Learning about this multiplicity has to be covert. This means that junior and student midwives have to discover it by working alongside and observing experienced midwives with learning being a form of 'we can know more than we can tell' (Polanyi 1966, p. 4). Hattie an independent midwife described her covert learning about the ways in which midwives could create 'grey area' in the following way:

You have midwives having ridiculous conversations where, you know, you're in there as the student saying 'oh I think she's fully dilated' and your midwife who's with you is saying 'oh she's probably got a bit of a lip' and [you're thinking] 'I'm sorry, I'm sorry, am I being a bit slow here?' (Laughs) 'Am I supposed to say she's got a bit of a lip?' You know, I'm thinking 'this is mad, this is mad …'. (Study I)

It is clear that while midwives actively endorse the prescribed evidence approach to practice in which their actions in relationship to labour such as vaginal examinations are oriented to and controlled by the official timetable embedded in the partogram, there exists an alternative approach to practice in which individual midwives use their professional judgement to subvert the timetable creating delay and space for labour to develop in its own time and own speed.

Discussion

As Brown *et al.* (2013) have noted, risk and time are inextricably linked. Risk involves the possibility of undesirable outcomes in the future and risk management involves minimising the possibility of such undesirable outcomes. Indeed, the development of risk and risk management can be link to the development of standardised and abstract time: time measured by mechanical and electronic devices, abstracted from and imposed on the rhythms of everyday lives of individuals and groups. For example, the influential Royal Society (1992) study report specified that an adverse event was one that occurred during a specified time period, by implication such a period must be one that can be measured and objectively defined. The emergence of such abstract time systems underpins the development of timetables where the future can be planned and plotted through standardised measures of time. Such timetables provided a mechanism for predicting and managing the future. The partogram timetable is designed to manage an uncertain future. By creating a time framework for labour, it enables midwives to categorise women as low or high risk and once women deviate from the partogram timetable and are categorised as high risk, they are seen as needing more surveillance and possibly medical intervention. Midwives tend to see the partogram as part of evidence-based practice that is it is based on systematic evidence from past cases. Risk categorisation becomes part of prescribed practice. Moreover, once they form part of practice, such categorisations become part of a self-fulfilling prophecy where women whose labour is delayed are treated as high risk and subjected to intervention associated with that categorisation. This self-fulfilling prophecy makes it impossible to assess whether or not the delay would have been associated with other negative outcomes had the medical intervention and risk recategorisation not taken place.

All the midwives in the study were aware of the importance of time in labour and largely accepted and worked within the partogram timetable – undertaking regular vaginal examinations as per protocol, recording in the partogram the progress of women's labour. However, occasionally midwives chose to disregard the timetable. Sometimes, the midwives in both of these studies deliberately misrepresented the results of their vaginal examination, for example, by recording 2–3 cm dilation when they felt it was actually 4–5 cm or indicating that there was a 'lip' so that the second stage had not started even though the cervix was fully dilated. In some cases, the timing of a mother's labour clashed with midwives own time, for example, full dilation coincided with the end of a shift and the midwife invented a lip so she could hand over the woman and finish her shift. However, more often midwives chose to do this because they felt that the partogram timetable imposed an artificial and potentially risky constraint on a woman's labour. They were confident in and preferred to rely on the signs and signals from the labouring woman's body. In these instances, embodied time was seen to exist outside of the partogram timetable, as a timeframe that deserved the midwife's attention. In some circumstances, the midwives felt that the prescribed timetable was too rigid. In such instances, the midwives justified covert activities explaining that they wanted to make it more flexible so that it would fit better with the woman's own body rhythm increasing the probability that the woman would have a spontaneous vaginal delivery and reducing the probability of what they saw as unnecessary medical intervention. Much of the midwives' observation was external, for example, frequency and nature of contractions or the noise and positions the mother favoured. However, to confirm their judgements, the midwives occasionally undertook extra vaginal examinations and since they had moved away from the official timetable and did not want to record the findings, some of these examinations were informal and undocumented 'quickies'.

The control and standardisation of the timing of clinical practice is a central part of clinical governance but rather than being an external managerial system, it has been presented as change managed and led by clinicians through the development of evidence-based practice. The shift involves a move from individual autonomous practice based on personal experience and intuition (embodied knowledge) to a collective control of work through guidelines and protocols (encoded knowledge). This collective control of practice involves a system in which clinical outcomes of individual clinicians (risks in the future) are monitored to ensure that they are based on agreed guidelines (decisions in the present) which are grounded in clinicians systematic reviews (evidence from the past). Harrison and Wood (2000) have described the shift in clinical practice in the following ways:

> [It] translates professional practice into a range of standardised procedures, workflows, protocols, templates and timescales, [and] aims to produce an audit trail against which key performance targets may be measured. (Harrison and Wood 2000, p. 26)

Midwives in both our studies accepted the logic and legitimacy of evidence-based practice and as we have noted they were hostile to and critical of practitioners who overtly and explicitly rejected this approach to practice. Thus, our findings support Brown and Crawford's (2003) view that health-care practitioners working in the NHS have 'become self-regulating "deep(ly) managed" subjects under a largely hands-off management regime' (p. 67). Far from suggesting that the midwives have not successfully internalised the scientific–bureaucratic timetable, we are simply suggesting that this internalisation should not be thought of as totalising. The midwives involved in these studies ostensibly sought to comply with the standardised behaviours expected of them by the encoded knowledge of the institutions in which they practiced. For example, they accepted the partogram timetable for managing labour, they undertook the prescribed vaginal examinations, recorded the findings on the partogram and summoned help when the labour exceeded the set time limits.

However, these same midwives were willing and able to engage in covert activities that undermined the timetable. In their day-to-day practice, the midwives involved in these two studies were balancing two divergent and concordant concerns with risk and time. On occasions, these midwives chose to understand the organisational protocols aimed at regulating and standardising time as a security against the low probability but high consequence risk of harm to the labouring woman and her baby. This understanding manifested itself in enthusiastic compliance with the organisation's risk management technologies. On other occasions conversely, these same midwives actively and creatively refuted and resisted those very same technologies as they were committed to reducing the risk of medical intervention, potentially high probability of potential of harm to mother and baby. This means that the managerial and policymaker's version of the organisation's activities were both realised and simultaneously unsettled through midwifery activity. Traynor (1996) presents a persuasive account of nursing staff agency, where improvisation at the point of service delivery operates to resist the Fordist underpinnings of scientific–bureaucratic styles of NHS management. Wells (1997) similarly presents empirical evidence to show how the operations of street-level bureaucracy, played out by NHS community mental health-care professionals, diverge away from the intentions of policymakers and managers. Ruston (2006) has more recently published an account of NHS nurses actively devising contingency techniques in order to subvert the strict practice algorithms of NHS Direct. In the midwifery literature, Weir (2006) has described this same sense of multiplicity in the meaning making and agency around how risk is perceived and acted upon in the USA. In short, there is a body of literature providing compelling evidence of how both acts of compliance with and resistance to risk technologies operate in conjunction within health-care provision, calling into question the totalising scope of the strictly regulated and audited risk management mechanisms of scientific–bureaucratic medicine.

In this article, we have provided new evidence of deep management as described by Brown and Crawford (2003), where professional discretion and traditional ideas such as intuition, co-exist, albeit awkwardly, with voluntary compliance to the organisational risk management technologies. Just as Lipsky suggested that 'low level decision making of street level bureaucrats' (2001, p. 84) operates to moderate management control and facilitate expressions of discretion, we want to point out that this street-level bureaucracy is itself tamed by an understanding that encoded forms of practice prevail within the maternity services. That is to say, the data we have used in this article indicate that any concordant ways of practice exist only at the edges of an otherwise omnipresent professional preoccupation with compliance with the technologies of scientific–bureaucratic health-care provision.

It is our contention in this article that the midwifery activity described operated to relocate the loci of risk towards the risk technologies themselves and the limitation imposed upon practice by those technologies. The instances described above indicate that in some contexts, practitioners grasp the opportunity to act upon a mutual and apparently pervasive understanding that the very technologies devised to mitigate the risks associated with birth through the strict management of time could be understood themselves as a site of significant, secondary risk. Inevitably, once this relocation of risk had taken place, the midwives involved tended to see it as their professional responsibility to devise mechanisms through which they could protect the mothers in their care and themselves from these perceived risks. Moreover, these devices had to be such that they could take place without detection from the institution's technologies of risk management. This is not to suggest that any of the midwives introduced in this article saw themselves as risk-takers. On the contrary, they saw their subverting endeavours as, on the one hand, a way of protecting the women in their care from the iatrogenic risks introduced through the strict application of the institutions risk/time technologies and on the other hand, a way of ensuring the system worked by protecting their own professional and personal interests.

Conclusion

The scientific–bureaucratic maternity service assumes a technical rational view of maternity care where the deliverer of a service, in this case the midwife, is thought to be someone who simply acts as a compliant agent for using encoded knowledge as it is set out in the institution's rules and guidelines under the auspices of the clinical governance agenda. By using ethnographic data, it has been possible to look at the multidimensional, complex and socially embedded processes involved in everyday midwifery activity in labour rooms in the UK. We have looked at how risk operates at different levels in midwifery discourse, some more covert than others, and therefore have been able to illustrate how cracks within the dominant risk paradigm operate to create space where other professional priorities can be, all be it tentatively, voiced.

In this article, we have explored the multiplicity of meaning and meaning making involved in midwifery-based street-level bureaucracy. By that we mean that while the midwives involved in this study generally saw the scientific bureaucracy of clinical governance as being good for client safety, at the same time they were constantly in the business of devising circumventing techniques. These midwives at once acquiesced to and opposed the clinical governance frameworks suggesting a state of reflexivity as much as compliance.

It is important to conclude that these concordant ways of knowing about risks, where clinical governance itself can be recast as a source of risk, should not be thought of as being oppositional in nature. Far from it. Not only does the evidence presented in this article demonstrate that midwives are not simply compliant or passive agents in the delivery of maternity care, it also suggests that their work at the margins of the risk functioned in unexpected ways. The proposition being made here is that the success of the scientific–bureaucratic approach to the maternity services depends, in part at least, upon covert activity where midwives express and act upon hidden knowledge where time can be reconsidered and measure through the usually quiet observation of a mother's body.

Note

1. 'Anterior lip' is a midwifery expression used to describe the final stages of the first stage of labour (the onset of regular painful contractions to full dilatation of the cervix). This expression refers to the neck of the womb and describes the baby's head has not having quite passed out of the womb into the vagina. Importantly, the mother is not expected to actively push out her baby until the anterior lip (or cervix) is no longer palpable on vaginal examination although evidence for this practice is weak.

References

Alaszewski, A., 2003. Risk, clinical governance and best value: restoring confidence in health and social care. *In*: S. Pickering and J. Thompson, eds. *Clinical governance and best value: meeting the modernisation agenda*. Edinburgh: Churchill Livingstone, 171–182.

Alaszewski, A. and Brown, P., 2012. *Making health policy: a critical introduction*. Cambridge: Polity Press.

Armstong, D., 1995. The rise of surveillance medicine. *Sociology of health & illness*, 17 (3), 393–404.

Bergstrom, L., *et al.*, 1992. 'You'll feel me touching you, sweetie': vaginal examinations during the second stage of labour. *Birth*, 19 (1), 10–18.

Brown, B. and Crawford, P., 2003. The clinical governance of the soul: 'deep management' and the self-regulating subject in integrated community mental health teams. *Social science & medicine*, 56 (1), 67–81.

Brown, P., Heyman, B., and Alaszewski, A., 2013. Time-framing and health risks. *Health, risk & society*, 15 (6–7), 479–488.

Bryman, A., 2004. *Social research methods*. 2nd ed. Oxford: Oxford University Press.

Department of Health, 1997. *The new NHS modern and dependable*. Cm 3807. London: HMSO.

Downe, S. and Dykes, F., 2009. Counting time in pregnancy and labour. *In*: C. McCourt, ed. *Childbirth, midwifery and concepts of time*. New York: Berghahn Books, 61–83.

Flynn, A., 2000. Clinical governance and governmentality. *Health, risk & society*, 4 (2), 155–170.

Groeschel, N. and Glover, P., 2001. The partograph used daily but rarely questioned. *Australian journal of midwifery: professional journal of the Australian college of midwives incorporated*, 14 (3), 22–27.

Gwyn, R., 2002. *Communicating health and illness*. London: Sage.

Harrison, S. and Wood, B., 2000. Scientific-bureaucratic medicine and UK Health Policy. *Review of policy research*, 17 (4), 25–42.

Lam, A., 2000. Tacit knowledge, organizational learning and societal institutions: an integrated framework. *Organisational studies*, 21 (3), 487–513.

Lavender, T., Hart, A., and Smyth, R., 2008. Effect of partogram use on outcomes for women in spontaneous labour at term. *Cochrane database of systematic reviews*, 8 (4), 1–22.

Lipsky, M., 2001. *Street-level bureaucracy: Dilemmas of the individual in public services*. New York: Russell Sage Foundation.

Naples, N., 2003. *Feminism and method: Ethnography, discourse analysis, and activist research*. New York: Routledge.

National Institute of Health and Clinical Excellence, 2007. Intrapartum care. Care of healthy women and their babies during childbirth. NICE Clinical Guideline 55. London: NICE.

Parker, M., 2007. Ethnography/ethics. *Social science & medicine (1982)*, 65 (11), 2248–2259.

Polanyi, M., 1966. *The tacit dimension*. London: Routledge and Kegan Paul.

The Royal Society, 1992. *Risk analysis, perception and management*. Report of a Royal Society Study Group. London: The Royal Society.

Russell, K., 2007. Mad, bad or different? Midwives experiences of supporting normal birth in obstetric led units. *British journal of midwifery*, 5 (3), 128–131.

Ruston, A., 2006. Interpreting and managing risk in a machine bureaucracy: professional decision making in NHS Direct. *Health, risk & society*, 8 (3), 257–271.

Scamell, M., 2011. The swan effect in midwifery talk and practice: a tension between normality and the language of risk. *Sociology of health & illness*, 33 (7), 987–1001.

Scamell, M. and Alaszewski, A., 2012. Fateful moments and the categorisation of risk: midwifery practice and the ever narrowing window of normality. *Health, risk & society*, 14 (2), 207–221.

Schmid, V. and Downe, S., 2010. Midwifery skills for normalising unusual labours. *In*: D. Walsh and S. Downe, eds. *Essential midwifery practice. Intrapartum care*. Oxford: Wiley-Blackwell, 159–190.

Shepherd, A. and Cheyne, H., 2012. The frequency and reasons for vaginal examinations in labour. *Women and birth*, 26 (1), 49–54.

Simonds, W., 2002. Watching the clock: keeping time during pregnancy, birth, and postpartum experiences. *Social science & medicine*, 55 (4), 559–570.

Stacey, J., 1988. Can there be a feminist ethnography? *Women's studies international forum*, 11 (1), 21–27.

Stewart, M., 2004. *Midwives discourse on vaginal examination in labour*. Thesis (PhD). University of the West of England, Bristol.

Stewart, M., 2005. 'I'm just going to wash you down': sanitizing the vaginal examination. *Journal of advanced nursing*, 51 (6), 587–594.

Traynor, M., 1996. A literary approach to managerial discourse after the NHS reforms. *Sociology of health & illness*, 18 (3), 315–340.

Walsh, D., 2010. Labour rhythms. *In*: S. Downe and D. Walsh, eds. *Essential midwifery practice: intrapartum care*. 1st ed. London: Wiley-Blackwell, 63–80.

Weir, L., 2006. *Pregnancy, risk and biopolitics*. London: Routledge.

Wells, S., 1997. Priorities, 'street level bureaucracy' and the community mental health team. *Health & social care in the community*, 5 (5), 333–342.

Pregnancy, risk perception and use of complementary and alternative medicine

Mary Mitchell[a] and Stuart McClean[b]

[a]Department of Nursing and Midwifery, University of the West of England, Bristol, UK;
[b]Department of Health and Applied Social Sciences, University of the West of England, Bristol, UK

Pregnancy and childbirth are events of major significance in women's lives. In western countries women are increasingly using complementary and alternative medicine during this time. However, there is little research exploring the factors that are influential in women's motivations to use complementary and alternative medicine during pregnancy and childbirth. This article draws on data from a narrative-based study designed to explore women's experiences of complementary and alternative medicine use during pregnancy and childbirth. The study involved 14 women living in the South-west of England, who had used complementary and alternative medicine during pregnancy and childbirth. We elicited narratives by interviewing women two to three times. The women in our study used complementary and alternative medicine both as a response to the uncertainty of pregnancy and childbirth and as a defence against manufactured risk, and in doing so indicated their desire to transform an unpredictable and unmanageable future into one which is more predictable and manageable. It was a means of dealing with the stress and anxiety associated with uncertainty which has to be dealt with. Their consciousness of the risks of biomedicine developed though the practice of complementary and alternative medicine, and their high educational status and relative affluence facilitated their choices. There was a tension evident in their narratives between a need to 'be in control' versus a desire for a natural childbirth without medical intervention. Women in the study showed their autonomy by actively pursuing complementary and alternative medicine while at the same time selectively using expert medical knowledge.

Introduction

Pregnancy and birth are pivotal experiences in women's lives with powerful personal and social significance. For most women pregnancy is a normal physiological process and in developed countries childbirth has a low probability of a harmful outcome. However, high expectations and the inevitable uncertainty of pregnancy outcomes have contributed to increasing medicalisation of birth with some arguing that modern childbirth is in crisis (Walsh 2006). Alongside this significant socio-cultural context, there is increasing evidence to suggest that pregnant women are increasingly using complementary and alternative medicine (Allaire *et al.* 2000, Hope-Allan *et al.* 2004, Mitchell and Allen 2008), a trend facilitated by the increased commodification of complementary and alternative medicine (McClean and Moore 2013). For the purposes of this article complementary and alternative medicine is defined as a range of health care practices which participants access outside of mainstream maternity services. The underpinning philosophies of these modalities are diverse, but mostly differ from biomedicine in their focus on the inter-connectedness of mind, body and spirit, the recognition of the power of the body to self-heal and the power of the therapeutic relationship (Kelner *et al.* 2003). Some research suggests that women utilise complementary and alternative medicine in pregnancy and birth in order to avoid the perceived 'risky' technological and pharmaceutical interven-tions associated with the medicalised approach to pregnancy management but empirical evidence of this is presently lacking (Smith *et al.* 2006, Mitchell and Allen 2008).

At the end of the nineteenth century and the early twentieth century there was increasing involvement of medical practitioners in birth, an increase in hospital birth and an increased use of technological interventions (Williams 1997). By the end of the 1970s a medical model of pregnancy and childbirth was firmly entrenched. In the 1990s, formalised risk management systems were introduced into the NHS, and the assessment, management and prevention of risks became the pivotal focus of the maternity services (Lankshear *et al.* 2005). Underpinning the biomedical approach is the view that pregnancy and childbirth are inherently dangerous, and therefore require medical supervision and technological interventions to ensure safe outcomes (Symon 2006). The laudable aim of risk management in maternity services is to improve the quality of care and patient safety (Heyman *et al.* 2010), yet this approach has contributed to the ever increasing rates of medical intervention in pregnancy and birth (Fenwick *et al.* 2010, Maier 2010). These practices are congruent with Beck's (1992) and Giddens' (1990) well-established thesis that risk and the management of risk have become increasingly important and pervasive in contemporary late-modernity.

In the UK less than two-thirds of women achieve birth without medical intervention and rates of operative birth are at an all-time high (BirthChoice UK 2012). Worry, anxiety and fear of childbirth is common and seems to be on the increase (Ayrlie *et al.* 2005), confirming a range of risk theorists' views about the fear generated by risk (Giddens, 1990, Beck 1992, Furedi 2002, Bauman 2006). Moreover, many women seem to have lost faith in their ability to birth naturally without medical intervention (Melender 2002, Hofberg and Ward 2003). As Davis-Floyd (2004) suggests the medical model shapes expectations, beliefs and practices and makes it difficult to think about pregnancy and birth in any other way.

In this article we draw on a recent empirical qualitative research which explored women's motivations to use complementary and alternative medicine, and the contribu-tion of complementary and alternative medicine to their everyday experience of pregnancy and childbirth. This article, considers the central issue of the utilisation of complementary and alternative medicine and the application of risk theory, in particular the concepts of reflexivity and fateful moments within the context of pregnancy and childbirth. The conceptual and theoretical context, which we discuss first, provides an important back-drop to key debates about the role of uncertainty in risk perception, and the role of agency in risk avoidance practices as women seek to manage risk by using complementary and alternative medicine during pregnancy and childbirth. We then discuss the aim and methodological approach of the study and then present the main findings of our narrative analysis.

Risk, pregnancy and childbirth: theorising the utilisation of complementary and alternative medicine

Social theorists such as Giddens (1990), Beck (1992) and others (Douglas 1992, Lash *et al.* 1996, Watson and Moran 2005) have highlighted the complexities of contemporary western societies in relation to a conceptual framework of risk. A common theme across these approaches is that risk has become increasingly important and pervasive in contemporary society. The 'risk society' is one in which the advantages of scientific and technological developments are overshadowed by risks and dangers, leading to anxiety and uncertainty (Beck 1992, Giddens 1990). A central motif is the everyday experience of living with risk, and yet despite the ubiquity of the conceptual framework, these theories have been neglected in the analysis of pregnancy, childbirth and the concomitant use of complementary and alternative medicine. Of particular interpretative relevance in our article is Beck's and Giddens' perspective on reflexivity and our analysis will centre on whether this concept can illuminate women's decision-making in choosing complementary and alternative medicine during pregnancy and childbirth.

Personal reflexivity is described by Beck (1996) as arising when individuals are faced with making decisions in the face of uncertainty. It includes critical reflection, self-confrontation and self-transformation as the anxieties and uncertainties about risk leads to a questioning of modern day practices. It refers to the self-authorisation of individuals, as they learn to negotiate contradictory discourses of science and expertise and exercise their autonomy in dealing with the problems and risks they face in everyday life. Beck and Giddens differ in their view of the relationship between risk and reflexivity. Beck's concept of reflexivity incorporates a critique of expert systems based on distrust, arguing that when individuals cannot trust experts or institutions they are compelled to seek their own solutions for problems they face (Beck 2009). Here the individual is viewed as making rational conscious decisions, weighing up the pros and cons of expert knowledge, and often developing their own areas of expertise. Other contemporary changes such as ease of access to information and the increasing desire of individuals for autonomy in decision-making help lubricate this process.

For Giddens (1990, p. 35) risk is consciously calculated, individuals make cognitive decisions but, in contrast to Beck, these are taken with a basic trust in institutions and experts. All actions of daily living require acceptance of advice from 'absent others', those unknown people or familiar institutions such as medicine, or the law (Giddens 1994, p. 89). Trust arises as a result of childhood experiences resulting in feelings of confidence or 'ontological security' in the reliability of people and social institutions. Ontological security provides an 'emotional inoculation' or 'protective cocoon' which leads to an attitude of hope and protects individuals against constant anxiety (Giddens 1991, pp. 39–40). A number of empirical studies confirm that notions of trust are central to risk perception and individual decision-making strategies (Green *et al.* 2003, Watson and Moran 2005, Brown 2009).

In Beck and Giddens' broadly realist position, risks are inescapable and thus individuals are compelled to confront, avoid or minimise risks. Although Beck (1999) is pessimistic about the risks of late modernity, he is optimistic about the power of social actors and agency in seeking creative solutions for themselves and in transforming social structures. Likewise, Giddens (1994) also highlights the power of individual agency as they actively create the social world around them rather than being determined by it (Tucker 1998).

However, socio-cultural dynamics underpinning risk perception seem more important in the analysis of risk perception in pregnancy. There is always the potential for danger to the mother and baby during pregnancy and childbirth. Nevertheless, women's perceptions and reactions to this risk vary and are often at odds with the professional discourses. The uncertainty and unpredictability of pregnancy and childbirth heightens women's feelings of vulnerability and loss of control. These feelings are congruent with Giddens' (1991, p. 131) description of 'fateful moments': as when 'an individual stands at the crossroads of his existence' (see also Scamell and Alaszewski 2012). Fateful moments precipitate a breach in 'ontological security' and intensify risk perception. Consequently, individuals adopt a variety of approaches to deal with these feelings of risk including denial. Being overly cautious: the 'precautionary principle' described by (Giddens 2002, p. 32) is one way in which individuals avoid difficult decision-making in the face of unknown risks and examples of this will be evident later in the article.

Perception of risk in pregnancy is complex and varied and is dependent on individual circumstances. Many women perceive low risk in pregnancy, but being aware of the uncertainty of pregnancy and birth are grateful for medical expertise and technology if and when it is required (Enkin 1994). Women who experience complicated pregnancies accept there is a risk to their own or their baby's health but their assessment of the magnitude of this risk may differ from that of the professional (Lee *et al.* 2012). For some women the perception of birth technology is equated with progressive medicine. Women request the use of electronic foetal monitoring in labour and access to pain relief at all times, and report these as essential for quality service (Green and Baston 2007). For some women, the risks of natural childbirth pose such fear they request elective caesarean section believing it is a safer option for themselves and their baby (Fenwick *et al.* 2010). Others reject all professional attendance during pregnancy and birth in the growing phenomenon of 'freebirthing' (Nolan 2008)

Such extremes reflect the social and culturally bound nature of risk argued by social theorists such as Douglas (1992) and Lash (2000). Women's reactions to risk thus highlight how perceptions of risk are inextricably linked with personal understandings of what constitutes a danger or a threat. Individuals often adopt complex and inconsistent strategies in dealing with risks, simultaneously displaying attitudes of trust, acceptance, rejection and scepticism (Giddens 1991, Adam *et al.* 2000). Bauman suggests (2006) that individuals are induced to search for biographical solutions to systematic and institutional problems. Women's use of complementary and alternative medicine during pregnancy and childbirth may be illustrative of this (Mitchell 2010, Lupton 1999). A number of studies have identified that pregnancy seems to provoke an increase in the use of complementary and alternative medicine (Allaire *et al.* 2000, Hope-Allan *et al.* 2004, Mitchell and Williams 2007). A number of factors have been shown to be influential in the use of complementary and alternative medicine during pregnancy and birth including dissatisfaction with biomedicine, concerns with the side effects of pharmaceuticals and a desire for more positive relationships with caregivers (Vincent and Furnham 2003). While the use of complementary and alternative medicine is increasing we currently have little understanding of why and how this relates to perceived risks of pregnancy and childbirth. In this article we aim to address this gap in evidence.

Methods: narrative research

Design

This article draws on an empirical study which used a narrative methodology to give voice to women's experiences of pregnancy and childbirth and their use of complementary and alternative medicine. Narrative research is an umbrella term that includes a wide variety of research approaches, which have at their heart individual stories (Elliott 2005). It is a genre within qualitative research which focuses on the meaning that individuals ascribe to life events (Czarniawska 2004). The importance of narrative enquiry lies in the notion that story telling allows individuals to make sense of their world, and that this process is retrospective in nature. This allows for an exploration of the meaning of important life events.

Narrative research does not aim to achieve explanatory power in recounting original experience since any recounting of events is subject to memory and is open to different interpretations (Atkinson's 1997). However, by acknowledging the social construction of the stories and through the telling and listening to stories it is possible to grasp the meaning of those experiences. The role of the researcher is to provide a level of interpretation that aids understanding of the phenomena under investigation. Knowledge claims made for narrative research need to be supported by strong and powerful arguments which allow for the presentation of meaning experienced by people (Polkinghorne 2007).

Sampling

We used a mixed sampling approach incorporating both purposive and snowballing strategies to identify a sample of women who had used complementary and alternative medicine during pregnancy and childbirth in the South-west of England. The sample was recruited by advertising through a local network of complementary and alternative medicine professionals. We did not use any incentives to aid recruitment as 14 women volunteered to take part in the study. These 14 women used a total of 20 different complementary and alternative medicine modalities between them during or following pregnancy. Their ages ranged from 30 to 49. One woman was from Germany, one Australian, one was Black American, one White American and the remainder were White British. All the women were in stable relationships. Educational status was high: all had further or higher education qualifications. Nine participants had used complementary and alternative medicine in their first and only pregnancy. The remainder had used complementary and alternative medicine in each pregnancy they had experienced, this ranged from 2 to 5. However, most women reflected on the use of complementary and alternative medicine during pregnancy and birth occurring within the past 1–2 years.

Data collection and analysis

In-depth interviews were conducted on two or three occasions with the 14 participants. The time frame that had elapsed since participants' complementary and alternative medicine use during pregnancy and birth varied from 6 weeks to 23 years. All but one of the interviews took place in the participants' homes. Most interviews lasted about 1.5 hours, the longest for 3 hours. Reissman (2008) suggests that understanding is achieved by encouraging people to describe their world in their own terms. *Tell me how you first became interested in complementary therapies* was the opening question for each participant. A desire to listen to their stories about pregnancy and birth was reflected by asking participants directly to *tell me about your pregnancy* or *tell me about your labour and birth*. Most, but not all women, completed their story to the present time in the first interview. The second and third interviews served as an opportunity for women to either continue telling their story or for the interviewer to question and seek clarification. A transcript of the first interview was made available to participants prior to subsequent interviews. Permission to undertake the study was granted by the University of the West of England, Faculty Research Ethics Committee on 4th August 2009.

Mary Mitchell transcribed the entire interview verbatim aiming to provide a full and faithful transcription. The interviews were analysed using a four-stage reading process informed by key proponents of narrative research such as Somers (1994) and Reissman (2008). We modified it with the intention of identifying the motivations, experiences and meaning of complementary and alternative medicine use. Reading 1 focussed on the narrative in its entirety as we were interested in the individual and their journey to the present day. In the second reading we identified the themes within and across participants' narratives. At the completion of this we identified sub-themes and core narratives and organised these using the computer software Nvivo. In reading 3 we focused on the analysis of discrete stylistic or linguistic characteristics of the narrative. In reading 4 we concentrated on socio-cultural influences in the narratives. The findings are presented in themes that were common across all participants. Both authors conducted the analysis and agreed on the emerging themes and interpretation of these in relation to risk theory. The final themes were shared with participants and feedback requested. To protect the identity, participants chose their own pseudonym.

Findings

In this section we highlight some of the findings of the study, focusing particularly on women's decisions to use CAM as a response to the uncertainty of pregnancy, their anxieties about risk and medicalised approach of standard maternity care. Where appropriate we will highlight the use of a conceptual framework of risk with reference to key theoretical approaches.

Pregnancy, 'fateful moments' and complementary and alternative medicine

For the participants in the study, pregnancy signalled a period of transition, a change in relationships and feelings of vulnerability. They talked about the unexpected impact of pregnancy on their emotions and shared their feelings of anxiety and vulnerability. One of the participants, Clarissa, explains the origins of her vulnerability:

> now I feel somehow more vulnerable than ever before, about life and your whole existence and it's just ... all of a sudden, it wasn't just about me, it was about somebody else and you have to think about somebody else and what that means....yeh definitely nerve racking. (Clarissa)

These feelings of vulnerability match Giddens' (1991, p. 131) description of 'fateful moments' and for participants precipitated a breach in 'ontological security'. Clarissa's comment *that everything changes*, the questioning of her *whole existence* and how she experiences having to *think about someone else now* highlighted the potential for pregnancy to threaten ontological security and to puncture the protective cocoon that usually filtered out anxieties about risks and dangers. This breach of ontological security generated anxiety and stress.

Feelings of vulnerability were amplified by the uncertainty of pregnancy. The potential for risk and for the development of unforeseen events was always considered a possibility. Women worried about their health and that of their baby, they worried about their ability to cope during labour and the risks of medical intervention. Participants had high expectations for their births so the antenatal period became a time to prepare and strengthen the body in anticipation of labour and their hope for normal birth. The uncertainty of how labour would progress and the inability to predict the outcome motivated women in their desire to be prepared for what they might face. This uncertainty had a profound effect on women. The resulting fear and anxiety impacted on their confidence to birth and prompted participants to seek a range of complementary and alternative medicine modalities which offered a sense of security and a way of influencing the future. A philosophy of active participation and preparation in order to strengthen the body, mind and spirit for the work of labour was integral to all the therapies women engaged in. As Riley noted:

> all of it (complementary and alternative medicine) was motivated by my desire to have a home birth and to have myself emotionally and physically prepared as possible.

Ironically, although the women in the study subscribed to the belief in the naturalness of childbirth, it was also seen as something that had to be anticipated, planned and prepared for as Caroline stated.

> I felt it was a real challenge like running a marathon. It was something I was preparing more mentally for 9 months and I wanted to do everything in my power to experience a natural birth. (Caroline)

Practices such as yoga and hypnobirthing were designed to help women develop self-help techniques of breathing, distraction, visualisation and positions to adopt in labour and provided the opportunity to practice these techniques. Thus, women in the study used these techniques to explore what labour might be like and how their actions could help them cope with the pain of labour. As Caroline explained *it* [yoga and hypnobirthing] *is like a rehearsal for childbirth*. However, despite all the preparations women undertook, there was always an undercurrent of fear and uncertainty that events may be unforeseen. Women turned to complementary and alternative medicine to help deal with these emotions. Riley said:

> I knew exactly what I wanted but it is also scary to know it might not happen. I know how easy it is not to happen and I didn't want to set myself up as horribly disappointed. I was investing a lot into how I wanted my labour to be. I was going to yoga every week, I was having acupuncture once a week and reflexology with a friend and then I saw a kinesiologist (Riley)

Media portrayal of childbirth partly contributed to their general anxiety and fears about childbirth as Daisy noted: *I have always been frightened about giving birth especially what you see on the TV and how it's a scary thing*. She attended antenatal yoga classes which provided her with the opportunity to be with women who hold a different perspective on birth as she explained:

That class was very much about pregnancy being a natural experience and not something to be frightened about and how it can be over medicalized. It took me from being frightened about childbirth to thinking of it in a completely different way. (Daisy)

Stephanie too harboured a deep fear of childbirth. A childhood experience of a sex education video left Stephanie *traumatised*. Erin reflected on the fact that it is difficult for women to tell positive birth stories for fear of being *smug or self-satisfied* and that there seems to be *something in connecting with other people through a shared trauma which means that those are the stories that get circulated*. Becker (1999) would agree that distress seems to be the major organising factor in the way life stories are told. Pregnant women were only exposed to stories of difficult and traumatic births. Attendance at group complementary and alternative medicine sessions meant women were in the company of other women with similar beliefs and desires to achieve a normal birth. Complementary and alternative medicine was influential in changing these participants' views about the naturalness of birth and their ability and confidence to birth in the way they had planned. Stephanie's use of acupuncture, hypnobirthing and hypnotherapy helped fundamentally change her beliefs about birth. She achieved the birth of two children in a community birth centre with no pain relief and described her experience as *just perfect*.

Becker (1999) argues people use cultural resources during times of vulnerability to help them make sense of their lives. Participants made reference to the accessibility of complementary and alternative medicine. Daisy talked about the normative culture of complementary and alternative medicine use in pregnancy:

My yoga class makes you feel you are not the only one and that it (complementary and alternative medicine) is an acceptable thing to do in pregnancy. (Daisy)

Thus, from early pregnancy many of the women in our study were immersed in a culture where complementary and alternative medicine was viewed as acceptable. For these women, using complementary and alternative medicine represented an attempt to re-establish the 'protective cocoon' of ontological security and signified a turning point in their lives as they learn to cope with their feelings of vulnerability and anxiety at this time.

Impact of risk discourses on the experience of pregnancy

The women in our study experienced anxiety and heightened sense of vulnerability in relation to their own health and that of their baby. Alison with children aged 23, 16 and 7 years old, was well placed to reflect on the impact of these risk-reduction strategies and the changes she had experienced over the years:

I find it really hard work since they have medicalized it [pregnancy and childbirth?] so much. When I had my first child (23 years ago) no one told you what to eat, what to drink and what to do. They were quite keen on giving up smoking, which was all they were worried about. By the time I was pregnant with ... (daughter age 16) you were not allowed to eat God knows how many different thing, liver, cheese, pate, no this, no that and then when I was pregnant with .... (son age 7) it was just even worse, you can't do this, you can't do that. I mean my Miriam Stoppard Mother and Baby book says relax in the evening with a glass of wine but by the time I had.... (son) if you had been drinking a glass of wine whilst breastfeeding the police would come in the door practically or they say there is a .0001 per cent chance this might happen so don't eat tuna, it's all risk.

Alison's narrative indicated the pervasiveness of risk practices in public health discourses which construct risk as a consequence of individual responsibility and life style choice (Gabe 1995, Lupton 1999). In following medical advice, the health of the baby takes priority and women's needs become subsumed by that of their foetus. For some of the women in our study complementary and alternative medicine was a *reward* or *treat* to make up for the hardships of pregnancy and for the lack of recognition of women's needs when the focus of care is on the well-being of the foetus. Alison described this in the following way:

> I think you have so much more need for that feeling of doing something for yourself because all the things that you used to do nice for yourself you are not allowed to do anymore because you are sacrificing yourself on the altar of this potential child. It's just nice to go off and have a massage. I think it's a reward for just being pregnant. (Alison)

Many of the women in our study experienced the so called 'minor disorders of pregnancy' but were reluctant to take standard biomedical treatments for fear of risks. Although Daisy said she knew that *paracetamol was safe* she would not take it to ease back-pain. Ladybird expressed a distrust of all mass produced products stating *God knows what they put in them!* Star's concerns reflected Beck's thesis of distrust in institutions and science and the consequential 'reflexivity of uncertainty':

> You don't actually know all the side effects, (of drugs) you don't know the long term side effects and you don't know what goes with what. They have got their double blind trials and whatever they want to prove but I think there are lots of risks and side effects, especially in pregnancy, what do you consider safe? (Star)

Star's narrative indicated that these women had to live in a world and make sense of these manufactured risks with the known and unknown side effects of drugs. As such the women had to make decisions knowing that some of the consequences were unforeseeable (Beck 1999). Daisy, Star and other women adopted the 'precautionary principle' (Giddens 2002, p. 32) avoiding drugs and their 'unknown' risks. Some of the women in the study were also cautious about using complementary and alternative medicine, for example, Daisy used chiropractic only because it *had been recommended by a midwife* as she would have *worried about it not being safe*. However most of the women in the study saw complementary and alternative medicine as safe and side effects perceived as minimal. This is in keeping with Slovic's (2000) argument that individuals exhibit a greater tolerance of self-imposed risks compared to those imposed by others. Women's previous positive experience of complementary and alternative medicine was the most important factor in their decision to use it during pregnancy. For example, Ladybird was familiar with the side effects of aromatherapy oils but from previous experience she *felt confident that it would be ok because my body is used to them.* Taking a risk then was different to being subjected to risks by others (Lyng 2008), in this way these women are exhibiting a desire for high levels of control and agency.

In their narratives, women in the study reflected on the ways in which pregnancy and childbirth are framed in terms of risk. They gave examples of how the care they received impacted on their worries and exacerbated anxieties about their health, that of their baby or their confidence to birth without medical intervention. Ladybird described how excited she was about attending her first antenatal appointment but the focus on risk left her feeling very scared:

> The very first appointment I had with the midwife was all about our family history and all the things which could go wrong. I found that very upsetting. I had gone from feeling extremely elated about being pregnant to being really scared that all these things could go wrong. (Ladybird)

As their pregnancies progressed, the women found the risk approach of maternity care increased their anxieties and fears. For example, Ladybird described how antenatal education classes reinforced the view that medical intervention in birth was the norm. A tour of the maternity unit served to increase her fears.

> when we went to do the tour of the hospital I came away feeling absolutely terrible, because I had never been to hospital before. It seemed very clinical and the tour finished outside the operating theatre and I was thinking well that's where I am going to end up. (Ladybird)

Riley described the ways in which her engagement with complementary and alternative medicine was an attempt to reduce anxiety about risk:

> they (complementary and alternative medicine) are an antidote to what is given to us which is a lot of fear. If we didn't live in a world where it is suggested that you can't have a baby without an epidural unless you are mad then you probably wouldn't need all of those things. Most people think you are kind of crazy to have a baby without pain relief or it's going to hurt so you would rather have a c. section. (Riley)

The women in the study described the ways in which complementary and alternative medicine practices such as hypnobirthing and yoga enabled them to prepare themselves for labour and birth in a way that fitted with their values and beliefs. Some participants chose complementary and alternative medicine as a way of supporting their desire for a normal birth one: without unnecessary medical intervention. For others, engagement with complementary and alternative medicine became a way of building their confidence and reducing their anxiety about the risks of giving birth.

CAM use as a reaction against routine medical intervention

Despite the extent of women's preparation for birth some participants found their plans and hopes for a normal birth thwarted before labour even commenced. For example, if labour had not commenced by 40 weeks (the medically defined period for full term), many women felt under pressure to accept a medical induction of labour.

> I suppose the threat of induction was fear about how induction can escalate into needing other drugs and things like that. That induction is forcing the body into something that it's not quite ready and then sets off a whole load of other problems whereas going into labour naturally seems to be, well you are ready for it, baby is ready for it. (Clarissa)

There is debate in the literature about the relative risks of prolonged pregnancy and of the induction process itself and there is lack of consensus about the best way of managing prolonged pregnancies (Westfall and Benoit 2004, Smith and Crowther 2008). Women in the study became aware of the discrepancy in professional advice, with some professionals recommending early induction of labour and others suggesting a more conservative approach or waiting for the onset of spontaneous labour. However, what is missing in the scientific debates about induction of labour is how *the threat of induction* impacts on a woman's belief about her ability to birth. When Clarissa did not go into spontaneous labour and she was offered induction, she began to question herself:

> I felt like I would have failed and I wasn't susceptible enough in my body or my body wasn't open, and under treat, under threat, that ... sort of motherhood thing, under threat because I will leave.... (baby) open to things or somehow making me feel not like a woman. It was really stressful trying to work out if we weren't just avoiding induction just because of this. (Clarissa)

The repetition of *threat* in Clarissa's narrative suggests the impact of medical discourses on her psyche, her femininity, as well as the concerns about physical risks to herself and her baby.

It seems for these women induction of labour had become a symbol of inappropriate medical intervention which threatened to undermine their philosophy of natural childbirth. Participants felt the threat *of induction* and subscribed to the belief that it is better for labour to start naturally. In the hope of getting their labour started rather than questioning the need to induce labour beyond term, women sought complementary and alternative medicine as a more natural means of instigating the onset of labour. Women in our study did not consider prolonged pregnancy to be a medical problem in itself but they felt pressurised by maternity carers to conform to standard policies and procedures. This is confirmed by other studies such as that of Westfall and Benoit (2004). Despite the clear policy agenda of informed choice set out in successive government reports such as Changing Childbirth (1993), Maternity Matters (2007) and the Choice Framework (DH 2012) research findings consistently show the rhetoric is not matched in reality. Institutional pressures, the contemporary discourses and professional language of pregnancy and birth act to limit the choice offered (Kirkham and Stapleton 2001, Scamell and Alaszewski 2012). When participants rejected the standard medical options they felt compelled to act, taking responsibility for their decisions and actions, as Caroline explained:

> they (doctors) have to tell me what the risks are but it's my decision. They are not held responsible if I chose not to go with the induction and he is stillborn. (Caroline)

Caroline's comment reflected the moral danger of going against medical advice. Viisainen (2000) suggests that such moral risks significantly impact on women's decision-making. For participants in this study complementary and alternative medicine provided emotional support and a way in which they could deal with the anxiety associated with this responsibility. Clarissa described the support she received from her homeopath:

> I saw the homeopath a few days after he was due and we looked at why that might be, so we started on homeopathic remedies. I was in contact with her every other day and then it became every day, just gently bringing things on. Seeing the homeopath and being in constant contact with her coming out of that meeting [with doctors] and speaking with her. She was just so encouraging with going along with how I felt as I was so scared to induce and then regret induction. (Clarissa)

Even though some women (Daisy, Alexandra, Stephanie, Ladybird and Riley) did not have prolonged pregnancy they did use a range of complementary and alternative medicine modalities such as reflexology, acupuncture and herbal products to encourage the onset of spontaneous labour and reduce the likelihood of induction. For this group of women, choosing complementary and alternative medicine modalities to support the onset of labour illustrates a backlash against routine medical approaches, and an attempt to take control of the situation and be active managers of their own pregnancies rather than being as Westfall and Benoit (2004) conclude 'disembodied subjects of medical intervention'. For these women the discourses of medicalisation and risk were powerful, opting out or resisting the advice of doctors and midwives provoked anxiety, fear and guilt (Heaman *et al.* 2004). Complementary and alternative medicine was a way to cope, and to reduce feelings of guilt by being proactive and as Rose described, *doing everything possible* to achieve the desired result.

For other participants, their desire for a normal birth was curtailed by the routine medical approach to managing birth, for example, when the baby lay in a breech position. Alison, Caroline and Ladybird sought complementary and alternative medicine when they found that their baby was in the breech position. When Rose's baby was discovered to be in a breech position she was devastated as she had planned a home birth. She was informed that *she would have to have a caesarean section*. Rose's immediate response was to reject this advice. She reflected on this choice as *obvious* as she was firm in her belief that there would be *another way to do it*. Determined to do everything she could to ensure a normal birth she practised specific physical exercises designed to facilitate the turning of the baby. She used meditation and visualisation: techniques learned from hypnotherapy and she sought treatment from an acupuncturist, an osteopath and a chiropractor but without effect. Subsequently, a routine medical procedure also failed and Rose had her baby by caesarean section. There is little evidence of reflexive calculation in Rose's behaviour and a sense of desperation was tangible in her frantic attempts to try as many therapies as possible to help achieve the home birth she desired. Rose explained she would try *anything if there was a chance it would help.* Sharma (2003) also refers to this notion of desperation in seeking complementary and alternative medicine. However, this rather negative connotation to complementary and alternative medicine has a different perspective as their actions contributed to their internal sense of identity, of being proactive and being in control. Reflecting on her experiences of complementary and alternative medicine Rose said:

> It makes you feel better doing it, you are thinking if there is a chance that this could work you should try it. I felt like I had done everything that I could, everything in my power. There is a part of you that thinks it might not work. It's just if you don't do it then how can you even know? (Rose)

The women in the study recognised the limitations of the 'scientific evidence' favoured by professionals. They appreciated the construction of scientific knowledge did not take into account personal or cultural circumstances and therefore they lacked trust in professional decisions. Caroline realised the ways in which broader societal pressures impacted on professional advice and professionals' articulation of risks:

> the culture of litigation is lurking there somewhere and they have to tell me what the risks are but it's my decision. (Caroline)

Discussion

The women in our study made decisions in a rational manner, weighing up the pros and cons of induction, reading widely, including accessing professional literature. Caroline, for example, knew the statistics for the increased risk of stillbirth in prolonged pregnancy. The women also incorporated into their decision-making strategies deeply held values and beliefs in relation, both a scepticism of expert knowledge and a belief and trust in their own bodies. Participants made decisions about complementary and alternative medicine that were relevant to their social and situational context. In many instances their actions could be described as both rational and irrational described by Zinn (2008) as an 'in-between' decision-making strategy in times of uncertainty. The practice of complementary and alternative medicine also the discourses of natural, the emphasis placed on listening to the body and the importance of 'being in control' all take place within the particular paradigm and epistemological beliefs of complementary and alternative medicine. The women in our study thus 'repositioned' risk within this framework.

Even though the women in our study did not necessarily accept expert assessment of risk, they had to make their decisions within the context in which risk was all-pervasive For these women the possibility of induction and unwanted medical intervention were omnipresent. They viewed induction or caesarean section as the catastrophic events they wanted to avoid at all costs. These women were forced to think about risk and as Beck has argued it is 'the staged anticipation of catastrophe obliges us to take preventative action' (Beck 1999, p. 90). Beck (1999) suggests in this kind of scenario, reactions frequently are of denial, apathy or transformation. However, the women in our study did not deny the risks or become apathetic instead they sought to transform their experience and manage the risk through complementary and alternative medicine.

For some of the women there was an aesthetic and hermeneutic dimension in their decision to use complementary and alternative medicine. Lash (2000) suggests that this aesthetic or hermeneutic reflexivity reveals itself in taste and style, consumption and leisure activities. Rather than seeking further medical advice or pharmacological treatment for anxiety, engagement in complementary and alternative medicine reflected this aesthetic and hermeneutic reflexivity. Other researchers have found too that the most valued elements of complementary and alternative medicine relate to aesthetic elements of comfort, touch, connection and caring (Smith *et al.* 2009). Hermeneutic reflexivity also involves emotion, intuition and imagination based on culturally acquired understandings. The role of imagination in decision-making may be particularly pertinent for pregnant women. Participants, having no other way of connecting with their baby, imagined the risk that their anxieties and fears may place on their well-being.

There are some limitations to the study which should also be considered in any interpretation. The sample was self-selected, relatively affluent and well educated, and all were enthusiastic complementary and alternative medicine users. Indeed, the women in our study spoke of their desire to take part in research to share their story of the positive contribution that complementary and alternative medicine made to their pregnancy and childbirth experience. Narratives can be disconnected and incomplete and thus have their limitations in revealing the very essence of experience (Richard 1997). Nevertheless, the findings illustrate how childbearing women negotiate perceived risks when deciding on how to manage their pregnancy and birth and their decisions to use complementary and alternative medicine.

In this article, we have shown that for the women in our study pregnancy was a 'fateful moment'. They indicated that they had a heightened sense of risk, uncertainty over pregnancy and birth outcomes, and fear of unwarranted medical interventions and that these feeling contributed to anxiety, worry, fear and sense of vulnerability. These feelings were a prime motivational factor in seeking complementary and alternative medicine. In participants' talk of stress and anxiety there was evidence of a breach in ontological security and an expressed need to re-establish the secure feelings of the 'protective cocoon' described by Giddens (1991, p. 40). With the failures of contemporary maternity care, participants found alternative ways to deal with their anxieties by seeking the relaxing effects of complementary and alternative medicine. Participants' anxieties and fears result from the uncertainty of pregnancy outcomes, the inevitable risks of pregnancy and birth and the potential risks of interventions. The focus on the assessment and management of physical risks of pregnancy on the mother and baby contrast sharply with the risks self-defined by women as lying within their emotional reactions and social domain. Finding a way to address these feelings became an imperative for participants' action in seeking complementary and alternative medicine.

Conclusion

Women's use of complementary and alternative medicine, whether as a response to the uncertainty of pregnancy and childbirth or as a defence against manufactured risk, reflected a desire to transform an unpredictable and unmanageable future into one which is more predictable and manageable. This supports Zinn's (2009) argument that we should focus on the ways in which individuals seek to manage uncertainty rather than risk: when outcomes are unpredictable or uncontrollable uncertainty assumes priority. It is the stress and anxiety associated with uncertainty which has to be dealt with. Participants demonstrated the critical reflexivity that Beck and Giddens refer to. Their growing consciousness of the risks of biomedicine developed though complementary and alternative medicine practice, aided by their high educational status and relative affluence facilitated their choices.

There was a tension evident in the women's use of complementary and alternative medicine and their underlying discourse for the need to 'be in control' versus their desire for a natural childbirth without medical intervention. The women in this study demonstrated their autonomy by actively pursuing complementary and alternative medicine but also engaging selectively with expert scientific knowledge.

Participants' decisions to pursue complementary and alternative medicine demonstrated the type of cognitive reflexivity described by Beck and Giddens, but more importantly reflexive decisions were based on emotion, intuition and aesthetics. In this article we have shown that the ontological insecurity of pregnancy and reflexivity which emerges during fateful moments motivates women to use complementary and alternative medicine. Women described the ways in which they used complementary and alternative medicine in this situation to retain control of their bodies and lives.

References

Adam, B., Beck, U., and Van Loon, J., 2000. *The risk society and beyond: critical issues for social theory.* London: Sage.

Allaire, A.D., Moos, M.K., and Wells, S.R., 2000. Complementary and alternative medicine in pregnancy; a survey of North Carolina midwives. *Obstetrics and gynaecology*, 95 (1), 19–23.

Atkinson, P., 1997. Narrative turn or Blind Alley? *Qualitative health research*, 7 (3), 325–344.

Ayrlie, G.M., Kethler, U., and Lohmann, S., 2005. Which components are important aspects of well-being in pregnancy. *MIDIRS midwifery digest*, 15 (2), 187–193.

Bauman, Z., 2006. *Liquid fear.* Cambridge: Polity Press.

Beck, U., 1992. *Risk society, towards a new modernity.* London: Sage.

Beck, U., 1996. Risk Society and the provident state. *In*: S. Lash, B. Szerszinksi and B. Wynne, eds. *Risk, environment and modernity: toward a new ecology.* London: Sage.

Beck, U., 1999. *World risk society.* Cambridge: Polity Press.

Beck, U., 2009. *World at risk*. Cambridge: Polity Press.

Becker, G., 1999. *Disrupted lives: how people create meaning in a chaotic world*. Berkeley, CA: University of Chicago Press.

Brown, P.R., 2009. The phenonemonology of trust: a schutzian analysis of the social construction of knowledge by gynaecology patients. *Health, risk & society*, 11 (5), 391–407.

Czarniawska, B., 2004. *Narratives in social science research*. London: Sage.

Davis-Floyd, R.E., 2004. Let me tell you a story. *The practising midwife*, 7 (6), 18.

Department of Health, 1993. *Changing childbirth*. London: HMSO.

Department of Health, 2007. *Maternity matters: choice, access and continuity of care in a safe service*. London: The Stationery Office.

Department of Health, 2012. 2013/14 Choice framework [online]. London: Department of Health. Available from: https://www.wp.dh.gov.uk/publications/files/2012/12/2013-14-Choice-Framework.pdf [Accessed 28 April 2013].

Douglas, M., 1992. *Risk and blame: essays in cultural theory*. London: Routledge.

Elliott, J., 2005. *Using narrative in social research, qualitative and quantitative approaches*. London: Sage.

Enkin, M., 1994. Risk in pregnancy, the reality, the perception and the concept. *Birth*, 21 (3), 131–134.

Fenwick, J., *et al.*, 2010. Why do women request caesarean section in a normal healthy first pregnancy. *Midwifery*, 26 (4), 394–400.

Furedi, F., 2002. *The culture of fear*. London: Cassells.

Gabe, J. ed., 1995. *Medicine health and risk*. Oxford: Blackwell.

Giddens, A., 1990. *The consequences of modernity*. Cambridge: Polity Press.

Giddens, A., 1991. *Modernity and self-identity*. Cambridge: Polity Press.

Giddens, A., 1994. Living in a post-traditional society. *In*: U. Beck, A. Giddens and S. Lash, eds. *Reflexive modernisation: politics, tradition and aesthetics in the modern social order*. Cambridge: Polity Press.

Giddens, A., 2002. *Runaway world: how globalisation is reshaping our lives*. London: Profile Books.

Green, J. and Baston, H., 2007. Have women become more willing to accept obstetric intervention and does this influence birth outcome? *Birth*, 34 (1), 6–13.

Green, J.M., Draper, A.K., and Dowler, E.A., 2003. Short cuts to safety: risks and rules of thumb in accounts of food choice. *Health, risk & society*, 5 (1), 33–52.

Heaman, M., Gupton, A., and Gregory, D., 2004. Factors influencing pregnant women's perceptions of risk. *Maternal and child nursing*, 29 (2), 111–116.

Heyman, B., *et al.*, 2010. *Risk, safety and clinical practice: health care through the lens of risk*. Oxford University Press.

Hofberg, K. and Ward, M.R., 2003. Fear of pregnancy and childbirth. *Postgraduate medical journal*, 79 (935), 505–510.

Hope-Allan, N., *et al.*, 2004. The use of acupuncture in maternity care: a pilot study evaluating the acupuncture service in an Australian hospital antenatal clinic. *Complementary therapies in nursing and midwifery*, 10 (4), 229–232.

Kelner, M. *et al.*, eds., 2003. *Complementary and alternative medicine, challenge and change*. London: Routledge.

Kirkham, M. and Stapleton, H., 2001. Informed choice in maternity care: an evaluation of evidence-based leaflets (CRD Report) [online]. York: Centre for Reviews & Dissemination, University of York NHS. Available from: http://www.york.ac.uk/inst/crd/CRD_Reports/crdreport20.pdf [Accessed 9 April 2013].

Lankshear, G., Ettore, E., and Mason, D., 2005. Decision-making, uncertainty and risk: exploring the complexity of work process in NHS delivery suites health. *Risk and society*, 7 (4), 361–377.

Lash, S., 2000. Risk Culture. *In*: B. Adam, U. Beck and J. Van Loon, eds. *The risk society and beyond critical issues for social theory*. London: Sage.

Lash, S., Szerszynski, B., and Wynne, B., 1996. *Risk, environment and modernity towards a new ecology*. London: Sage.

Lee, S., Ayers, S., and Holden, D., 2012. Risk Perception of women during high risk pregnancy: a systematic review. *Health risk and society*, 14 (6), 511– 531.

Lupton, D., 1999. *Risk*. London: Routledge.

Lyng, S., 2008. Edgework, risk and uncertainty. *In*: J.O. Zinn, ed. *Social theories of risk and uncertainity*. London: Blackwell

Maier, B., 2010. Women's worries about childbirth: making safe choices. *British journal of midwifery*, 18 (5), 293–299.

McClean, S. and Moore, R., 2013. Money, commodification and complementary healthcare: theorising personalised medicine with depersonalised systems of exchange. *Social theory and health*, 11, 194–214.

Melender, H., 2002. Experiences of fears associated with pregnancy and childbirth: a study of 329 women. *Birth*, 27 (3), 101–111.

Mitchell, M., 2010. Pregnancy, risk, and complementary therapies. *Complementary therapies in clinical practice*, 16 (2), 109–113.

Mitchell, M. and Allen, K., 2008. An exploratory study of women's and key stakeholders experiences of using moxibustion for cephalic version in breech presentation. *Complementary therapies in clinical practice*, 14 (4), 264–272.

Mitchell, M. and Williams, J., 2007. The role of midwife-complementary therapists: data from in depth telephone interviews. *Evidenced based midwifery*, 5 (3), 93–99.

Nolan, M., 2008. Free birthing: why on earth would women choose it? *The practising midwife*, 11 (6), 16–18.

Polkinghorne, D.E., 2007. Validity issues in narrative research. *Qualitative inquiry*, 13 (3), 471–486.

Richard, L., 1997. *Fields of play*. New Brunswick, NJ: Rutgers University Press.

Riessman, C.K., 2008. *Narrative methods for the Human Sciences*. Los Angeles, CA: Sage.

Scamell, M. and Alaszewski, A., 2012. Fateful moments and the categorisation of risk: midwifery practice and the ever narrowing window of normality during childbirth. *Health, risk & society*, 14 (2), 207–221.

Sharma, U., 2003. Medical Pluralism and the future of CAM. *In*: M. Kelner, *et al.*, eds. *Complementary and alternative medicine, challenge and change*. London: Routledge.

Slovic, P., 2000. *Perception of risk*. Sterling, VA: Earthscan.

Smith, C.A., *et al.*, 2006. Complementary and alternative therapies for pain management in labour. *Cochrane Database of Systematic Reviews*, 18 (4), CD003521.

Smith, C.A. and Crowther, C.A., 2008. Acupuncture for induction of labour. *Cochrane Database of Systematic Reviews*. doi:10.1002/14651858.CD002962.pub2

Smith, J., Sullivan, J., and Baxter, D., 2009. The culture of massage therapy: valued elements and the role of comfort, contact, touch, connection and caring. *Complementary therapies in medicine*, 17 (4), 181–189.

Somers, M.R., 1994. The narrative construction of identity: a relational and network approach. *Theory and society*, 23 (5), 605–649.

Symon, A., 2006. *Risk and choice in maternity care: an international perspective*. Edinburgh: Churchill Livingstone.

Tucker, K.H., 1998. *Anthony Giddens and modern social theory*. London: Sage.

Viisainen, K., 2000. The moral dangers of home birth: parents' perceptions of risks in home birth in Finland. *Sociology of health and illness*, 22 (6), 792–814.

Vincent, C. and Furnham, A., 2003. Users of CAM. *In*: M. Kelner, *et al.*, eds. *Complementary and alternative medicine, challenge and change*. London: Routledge.

Walsh, D., 2006. Risk and normality in maternity care: revisioning risk for normal childbirth. *In*: A. Symon, ed. *Risk and choice in maternity care*. Edindurgh: Churchill Livingstone.

Watson, S. and Moran, A. eds., 2005. *Trust, risk and uncertainty*. Hampshire: Macmillan.

Westfall, R.E. and Benoit, C., 2004. The rhetoric of 'natural' in natural childbirth childbearing women's perspectives on prolonged pregnancy and induction of labour. *Social sciences and medicine*, 59 (7), 138–140.

Williams, S.A., 1997. *Women and childbirth in the 20th century stroud*. Stroud: Sutton Publishing.

Zinn, J.O., 2008. A comparison of sociological theorising on risk and uncertainty. *In*: J.O. Zinn, ed. *Social theories of risk and uncertainty: an introduction*. Oxford: Blackwell.

Zinn, J.O., 2009. The sociology of risk and uncertainty a response to Judith Green's is it time for the sociology of health to abandon risk. *Health, risk & society*, 11 (6), 509–526.

Fateful moments and the categorisation of risk: Midwifery practice and the ever-narrowing window of normality during childbirth

Mandie Scamell[a] and Andy Alaszewski[b]

[a]Department of Midwifery, Florence Nightingale School of Nursing and Midwifery, King's College London, London, UK; [b]Centre for Health Services Studies, University of Kent, Canterbury, UK

In this article, we examine the ways in which risk is categorised in childbirth, and how such categorisation shapes decision-making in the risk management of childbirth. We consider the ways in which midwives focus on and highlight particular adverse events that threaten the normality of childbirth and the life of the mother and/or her baby. We argue that such a focus tends to override other elements of risk, especially the low probability of such adverse events, resulting in 'an ever-narrowing window of normality' and a precautionary approach to the management of uncertainty. We start our analysis with a discussion of the nature of childbirth as a fateful moment in the lives of those involved, and consider the ways in which this fateful moment is structured in contemporary society. In this discussion, we highlight a major paradox; although normal childbirth is both highly valued and associated with good outcomes in countries like the UK, there has been an apparent relentless expansion of 'the birth machine' whereby birth is increasingly defined through the medicalised practices of intensive surveillance and technocratic intervention. We explore the dynamics that create this paradox using ethnographic fieldwork. In the course of this work, the lead author observed and recorded midwives' work and talk in four clinical settings in England during 2009 and 2010. In this article, we focus on how midwives orientate themselves to normality and risk through their everyday talk and practice; and on how normality and risk interact to shape the ways in which birth can be legitimately imagined. We show that language plays a key role in the categorisation of risk. Normality was signified only through an absence of risk, and had few linguistic signifiers of its own through which it could be identified and defended. Where normality only existed as the non-occurrence of unwanted futures, imagined futures where things went wrong took on a very real existence in the present, thereby impacting upon how birth could be conceptualised and managed. As such midwifery activity can be said to function, not to preserve normality but to introduce a pathologisation process where birth can never be categorised as normal until it is over.

Introduction

In this article we focus on the ways in which midwives categorise risk in the context of childbirth. We start our analysis with a discussion of the nature of childbirth as a fateful moment in the lives of those involved, and consider the ways in which this fateful moment has changed and is structured in contemporary society. In this discussion, we highlight a major paradox; although normal childbirth is both highly valued and associated with good outcomes, there has been an apparent relentless expansion of 'the birth machine' (Wagner 1994), where birth performance is increasingly defined using medicalised practices of intensive surveillance and technocratic intervention. We then argue that the only way to understand this paradox is through fieldwork that captures the ways in which midwives make decisions during the birthing process. In the main part of this article, we will draw on fieldwork data to explore how midwives' talk and practice structure risk and normality.

Contemporary childbirth: Midwifery, normality and risk

Childbirth can be seen as a fateful moment in which life is changed irreversibly. If all goes well, then a healthy baby is born. But if things go wrong, then the mother and/ or her baby can be seriously harmed or even die. All those involved in a birth of baby *'must launch out into something new, knowing that a decision made, or a specific course of action followed, has an irreversible quality, or at least that it will be difficult thereafter to revert to the old paths'* (Giddens 1991, p. 114).

In premodern societies, interventions in childbirth were limited with little proven efficacy, so that the outcomes were, from a modern perspective, the product of chance. Though most mothers and their babies survived childbirth, there was a relatively high probability of adverse outcomes in comparison to today. Loudon (1993) estimated that in the early eighteenth century, 1000 women died for every 100,000 births. The death of babies is difficult to calculate as historic records are limited and inaccurate. However Davenport's (n.d.) study of records for London in the eighteenth century suggested an average of 30 stillbirths per 1000 births. Her more detailed study of the parish records of St Martin-in-Fields indicated around 60 deaths per 1000 in this location, with the rate fluctuating over the century between 40 and nearly 100 deaths per 1000 births. Thus, in eighteenth century London, based on the St Martin's figures, there was a .06 probability that the baby would not survive, and a .001 probability that the mother would not survive each birth.

In the twenty-first century, childbirth has become a vastly safer process in developed countries. The probability of dying during pregnancy and childbirth has fallen substantially. The Centre for Maternal and Child Enquiries (2011) indicated that, in the three years 2006–2008, only 261 women in the UK died as a result of their pregnancy, and that 4.67 deaths per 100,000 pregnancies could be directly attributed to the pregnancy including the childbirth. The stillbirth rate has also declined substantially, to 5.2 per 1000 births in 2007 (Confidential Enquiry into Maternal and Child Health 2009, p. 3). Thus, in countries like the UK, childbirth has become a much safer process.

However increasing safety is not the only difference between traditional and modern childbirth. There is also increase in human agency and choice. Traditional childbirth can be seen as a natural process in so far as lack of knowledge and skills limited human capacity to influence the outcome. Women giving birth had to cope with and manage the uncertainty of the outcome using such resources as were available to them.

The growth of scientific knowledge has radically changed the nature of childbirth in contemporary society, and provides the basis for expert risk management. Such expertise has transformed the capacity for informed decision-making through the application of human agency to change the probabilities of outcomes. Risk is now central to the 'rational' management of uncertainty. Since the end of the nineteenth century, all childbirth in the UK has been under the state-sanctioned surveillance of experts. In the UK and elsewhere, the type of surveillance used depends on expert classification of risk. Births by 'low risk' mothers can be supervised by midwives, and take place in low tech facilities, even in the mother's own home. Births by 'high risk' mothers should be supervised by obstetricians and take place in high-tech facilities. Despite this, however, high risk birthing environments continue to be the most the most used setting for the majority of mothers in the UK, with 88.2% of births in England taking place within an obstetric-led facility in 2010–2011 (NHS Health and Social Care Information Centre 2011a). In high-tech units, obstetric surgeons can, as a last resort, use a caesarean section to remove the baby from its mother's womb. The modern use of sections started in the late nineteenth century, and is now routinised in many health care systems. In the UK, the average caesarean section rate for both 2007–2008 and 2008–2009 was 24.6% (The Health and Social Care Information Centre 2009).

The development of scientific knowledge, and with it the capacity to make decisions that influence the outcome of the birthing process in the way intended, has altered the status of birthing attendants. They have become responsible and accountable for their decisions. Birthing is no longer a purely 'natural' process in which the outcomes are the product of chance and adverse outcomes are unpreventable 'accidents'. It is increasingly viewed as 'man-made', and therefore adverse outcomes cannot be accidental – see Green (1999) for an analysis of ways of the ways in which risk has eroded the concept of the accident – but must be the fault of those who made the decisions. As Douglas (1990) has argued, the concept of risk underpins the development of a 'blame culture' in which all harmful events are seen as a product of human agency, and every misfortune is someone's fault. She argues that '*under the banner of risk reduction, a new blaming system has replaced the former system based on religion and sin*' (Douglas 1992, p. 16).

Since the probability of actual harm to the mother or the baby (such as massive haemorrhage or significant birth asphyxia) during the process of spontaneous birth is small, midwives should be able to treat mothers as being capable of birthing their offspring without undue concern for risk. Indeed, midwives in the UK describe themselves as practising within a paradigm of normality (Gould 2000, Sandall *et al.* 2009, Midwifery 2020). Within this framework, women and their pregnant bodies are conceptualised as being essentially competent. Such a framework positions the midwife as a facilitator whose professional understandings of the spontaneous physiological process of birth can be applied through practice to ensure that babies are born with as little disturbance and intervention as possible (Rosser 1998, Leap 2000). Midwifery discourse tends to privilege notions of birth as a normal process (Davis-Floyd *et al.* 2009).

It follows that the categorisation of birth as high risk should be rare and exceptional. However, as we noted above, in practice the majority of births in England take place within a high risk birthing facility regardless of the risk status attributed to the pregnancy (NHS Health and Social Care Information Centre 2011a). There are two principal ways in which the decision to categorise a birth as high risk can be taken. Before the birth starts a midwife may judge that a mother has certain characteristics that place her in the high risk category, for example, if she is above a specified age when having her first baby. Alternatively, the decision may be made during the birth process when events do not follow the normal (and prescribed) trajectory, for instance, if the dilation of the cervix falls outside the 'normal' range. In this paper we will focus on this second type of high risk categorisation.

In this article, we explore why midwives who are committed in principle to normal childbirth are unable to articulate and defend normality. Instead, they often highlight the dangers of birth, creating the medicalisation of birth by categorising an increasing proportion of births as high risk. The paradox which we focus on was articulated by Carina, a midwife who participated in our study, in terms of 'what seems to be an ever-narrowing window of normality' (extract from interview with Carina, midwife).

Methods: Using ethnographic methods to access midwives' practice and the tacit knowledge which underpins them

This paper is based on data drawn from an ethnographic study designed to explore how midwives make sense of risk. In this study, we used methodological tools that could make explicit midwives' tacit knowledge, their common-sense understandings about risk and normality. The aim of the research was to observe and record situated midwifery talk and practice in the various clinical settings in which midwives work. The most effective way to access such activity was for the lead author (a qualified midwife) to participate in and observe birthing in different settings. This ethnographic approach was not employed in the early anthropological, positivist sense, as an attempt to capture what was 'really out there'. Instead the lead author adopted a reflexive approach in which her identity as a midwife and a researcher was implicitly woven into the process of data collection, and also shaped the production and analysis of an ethnographic text.[1]

To observe midwifery practice and talk in different settings, we selected four very different settings that represent the major organisational forms for birthing and midwifery practice in the UK. These settings were: a obstetric-led unit with all the medical facilities for high risk births (3361 births per year); two midwife-led units, one located in a hospital with access to back-up medical facilities in case a birth shifted from low to high risk category (606 births per year); a free standing midwifery-led birthing unit where the reclassification of a birth into the high risk category involved a 40-minute transfer journey (378 births per year) and, finally, a home birth service (224 births per year).

For this study, we used ethnography in its broadest sense, not so much as a set of research methods or analysis techniques, but as a 'concern with the meaning of actions and events to the people we seek to understand' (Spradley 1980, p. 5). As such, we considered the methods to be the most effective for achieving our desired objective – understanding situated midwives' meaning-making. As the fieldwork and associated analysis developed, we adapted, adopted or, in some cases suspended, various research tools (Clifford and Marcus 1986, Denzin 1998, 2002). Thus, our emphasis approach changed, depending on the issues raised by the data analysis, and included a combination of:

- participant observation (Malinowski 1932, Spradley 1980) ($n=42$) of midwifery labour care with midwives of various levels of seniority and in various care settings in order to observe what actually happens in practice
- non-participant observation ($n=15$). This was mainly done in 'behind the scenes' National Health Service (NHS) observations, such as board meetings,

staff meetings, protocol meetings and risk case reviews at unit and trust level, to gain insight into organisational issues which constrain and facilitate different kinds of practice

- ethnographic interviews (Spradley 1979) with managers, midwives, students and maternity and midwifery pressure group members ($n = 27$),[2] which allowed for the testing of hypotheses and the scrutiny of incidents observed during participant observation
- text analysis (Fairclough 2001, 2003) of protocols, policy documents and key professional texts to give a broader social and cultural contextualisation to the observation and interview data.

Analysis

Since the main objective of the research was to access midwives' intuitive knowledge, the analysis involved a careful reading and content analysis of field notes, interviews and related texts (Reissman 1993, Graneheim and Lundman 2004). Ongoing analysis was carried out alongside, and guided, the fieldwork. Following an initial reading, we undertook closer scrutiny of the texts produced within the study using conversational and discourse analysis techniques (Silverman 1988, 2004, Van Dijk 1993, 1997, Fairclough and Wodak 1997, Wodak 1999, Fairclough 2001, Gwyn 2002). This initial content analysis was checked and corroborated through the project supervision process, and was then intensified towards the end of the research, using ATLAS.ti to check for reliability and validity of the analysis; codes were networked and checked for density to ensure groundedness. In this paper, we focus on the data relating two codes – 'normal birth' and 'risk'. These were both densely populated codes, although 'normal birth' was more complexly networked and denser than risk.

Access and ethics

We accessed the initial sample ($n = 33$) using a process of self-selection, following a recruitment and information campaign targeted at all midwives working in the selected sites; and then expanded participation through opportunistic, snowball techniques (Bryman 2004), with some attention to purposeful structuring to maximise diversity. We obtained written consent and sequential verbal consent from all those involved in the study, and 'cleaned' all transcripts and field notes by removing identifying features prior to analysis. We sought ethical approval from both national and local NHS ethics committees, and obtained full approval for the study in February 2009. The NHS Trust's Research and Development governance team, the Head of Risk, Assurance and Legal Services and the Head of Midwifery reviewed and approved the project before we started data collection. The lead author had a NHS licence to practice for the duration of the data collection.[3] All data published in this paper have been 'cleaned' to remove identifying features, and all names have been changed.

Findings: Evidence from midwifery practice and discourses

Adverse outcomes, blame and risk

The midwives who participated in our study were aware of their accountability, especially in relation to adverse outcomes. As Heather indicated, positive outcomes did not attract attention or praise, whereas adverse outcomes attracted both attention and blame:

> *Well you see, if the outcome was fine it would never really get questioned would it? If there was a poor outcome you would be asked, 'Why I did that?' Good outcomes, well they never get investigated or celebrated really for that matter, it's only the, the poor outcomes. They're what everyone hears about, they're the things that make people sit up and take notice, you see.* (Extract from interview with Heather, senior midwife)

While accountability and potential blame formed the backdrop for much of research, in some circumstances it was foregrounded. For example, the demeanour of one midwife changed radically during the research. When she first worked with the lead author, she was confident and bubbly. However, as the field notes indicate, following her involvement in an internal risk inquiry she lost confidence and self-belief:

> Helen kept reiterating that she was nervous, explaining that whereas she had felt clinically confident in the past, recent events had made her feel *'so shit'* that she was sometimes unable to make the simplest of decisions sometimes. The way she overcame her confidence crisis was to picture herself discussing the case with the consultant midwife – P. *'I know this must be okay'*, she told me, *'because this is what P would say. She would say she is not in labour so I know it's okay to treat her like this'*. Helen and I left the room (where a mother was labouring) so that Helen could discuss her care plan with another midwife who had just arrived at the unit. During our conversation, Helen revealed more details about the incident that seemed to be haunting her practice so much. Helen explained that she was not traumatised by the event itself, stressing, with tears in her eyes, that *'I know I didn't do anything wrong. I know I am a good midwife . . . [I] know we are told it is not a blame culture, but this thing has been all about blame . . . It makes you feel like a bloody criminal! This job can be so shit sometimes'*. (Extract from field notes HJ 4).

Although personal involvement in an incident and subsequent inquiry highlighted the way in which blame was allocated, those midwives with little direct experience of adverse outcomes and related inquiries were made aware, through activities such as staff training sessions, that such circumstances could happen to them one day.

Fateful moments and the risk of adverse outcomes

For both midwives and mothers, birth was a fateful moment, but what was at stake differed. The midwives who contributed to our study were aware of their accountability, and of the personal consequences associated with adverse outcomes. So, if the birth did not go to plan, then not only could the mother and baby be harmed, but also the midwife would also need to account for her actions in an inquiry which would start from the premise that errors had been made.

As Giddens (1991, p. 127) has noted, one way of managing the threat of uncertain outcomes is through denial. When risk is part of everyday activities, such as crossing a road or preparing and eating food, familiarity and habit enable individuals to deny or bracket out the threat, creating a protective cocoon of routine. For birthing mothers, one would expect the unusual and atypical nature of the event to puncture the protective cocoon of normality. However what is unusual and exceptional for most mothers, childbirth, should be normal and routine for qualified midwives. To be qualified and granted a licence to practice, they need to provide evidence that they have participated in at least 40 births. One might expect the normality and routineness of most childbirth to sustain a protective cocoon for midwives (see Menzies 1960, for a discussion of the routines and structures in general nursing as defences against anxiety).

The fieldwork produced little evidence for the presence of a protective cocoon of routine. Midwives indicated that in their practice they were always alert to the possibility of adverse outcomes:

> *We are very risk averse aren't we.? We, we will say, within the NHS, the majority will say it* [birth] *is normal after the event.* (Extract from interview with Susan, a senior midwife)

From this perspective, all births were potentially hazardous, and normality could only be recognised in hindsight, after a woman had given birth to her baby and was no longer in the crisis of labour. Interviews with midwives, including those who were senior and experienced, indicated that during childbirth imagined risk was ever-present in a future inhabited by potential adverse events. Such adversities which this 'normal in retrospect' lens highlighted did not necessarily have much connection to events in the present, especially the probability of such events. Rather, it reflected the 'high consequences' of these events. What was being bracketed out was not potential adverse consequences but another important component of risk, their (low) probability. Midwifery practice coalesced around an apparently irresistible desire to anticipate and avoid even the smallest possibility of an adverse outcome, even when this might involve abandoning any commitment to the notion of normality:

> Maria: *I always tell people that there is high risk and there is low risk but that there is no such thing as no risk ... Risk is much more important even if it might not be clinically significant ...*
>
> Researcher: *A 1:10,000 risk, is that a high risk or low risk?*
>
> Maria: *Depends if you are the one really doesn't it.* [Laugh]. (Extract from interview with Maria, midwife)

In the context of midwife practice and talk, low risk or normal birth, despite being a preferred outcome, appeared to have a limited temporal existence, in that it could only exist in the past, after the events of birth had concluded. The ways in which many of the midwives, particularly those in positions of authority, talked about birth indicated that fears about the possibility of things going wrong functioned to destabilise professional confidence in birth normality. Such anxieties were evident in several of the training sessions which the lead author attended, which often focussed on the ways in which things could and did go wrong:

> As I looked around the room many of the midwives in the group were grimacing in horror as the session unfolded. Furthermore, the coffee break which followed this session was spent exchanging and collaborating over stories of near misses where risks lay waiting to develop into future Confidential Enquiry statistics. (Extract from field notes SD1)

The risk paradox: Midwives' commitment to normality

The overshadowing of midwifery practice by imagined futures containing potential adverse events was paradoxical as much of their talk stressed the positive value of normal birth. Normality was consistently represented as a cultural 'good'. Its merits were simply taken-for-granted, and this view was so deeply engrained into their shared tacit knowledge that a positive moral loading of the term was common to all midwives whom the lead author spoke to. When participants talked to her about normality, they simply assumed that she, as a fellow midwife, would share their understanding and appreciation of the term and its virtues. Explicit explanation was therefore deemed irrelevant, even comical. A belief in normality as a cultural good was a basis for identity as a midwife, something to be aspired to, and a source of professional pride and confidence:

> *Midwives very often come into the profession because they are women and intrinsically that they understand that birth is a normal process.* (Extract from interview with Silvia, midwife)

To be a midwife was to have an undefined and indefinable belief in the possibility of normality in childbirth – a notion reminiscent of the act of faith that underpins trust. Furthermore, several of the midwives we spoke to suggested that normality and midwifery were symbiotically linked – one could recognise one through the presence of the other. And birth could remain 'normal' even if there was some (limited) physical intervention in the woman's body:

> *Mmm, things like a stretch and sweep[4] and using entonox[5] ... well they are all things done by a midwife aren't they, so I suppose that doesn't make the birth, you know, just because a woman has those sorts of things doesn't mean her birth isn't normal, does it? ... So yer, you can have midwifery care, midwifery care and normality are sort of ... well they go together really don't they? They are the same ... because you see, midwifery care is low risk care isn't it? Mmm ... and a vaginal birth, yer normal vaginal birth, and, hopefully, a natural third stage, physiological third stage, all the stuff that can be managed exclusively by a midwife.* (Extract from interview with Rachel, midwife)

Thus, for Rachael, midwifery practice was symbiotically linked to normal birth. The boundaries of normality were marked by autonomous midwifery intervention, described here as the administration of entonox and/or the undertaking of a 'stretch and sweep' for induction of labour. Midwifery activity, even when it is directed towards interfering with the physiological birth process or introducing pharmaceutical agents to disrupt the woman's experience of birth, coincided with normality to such an extent that they become virtually one in the same thing – a normal birth was a midwife-managed birth.

In midwife talk, the term 'normal birth' was frequently pre-fixed with 'nice'. This lexical choice had a normative function, confirming the speaker's professional allegiances, and emotionally defining normality as a professional good, an interpretive framework which the following field note entry illustrates:

In the nurses' station [on a busy obstetric lead labour ward], Emma, a midwife was giving a history of the woman she had been caring for in 'hand-over' when she told the oncoming day staff: '*Despite all that* [referring to a catalogue of difficulties the mother had encountered during her labour] we did manage to get a *nice* normal delivery.' The reaction of the other midwives whom this comment was aimed at was one of approval, even mild congratulation. Emma had done well – the fact that she had managed to 'get a nice normal delivery' reflected well on her midwifery skills. (Emphasis added. Extract from field notes E14)

Not only was '*normal*' pre-fixed with '*nice*'. In addition, the word '*managed*' in this context suggests that normal birth should be considered something of an achievement. Good midwifery and normality appear mutually dependent. Given that normality is a preferable outcome, and that normal birth is less hazardous, we need to consider why it is so difficult to protect in current midwifery practice.

The vulnerability of normality: Its absence in talk and practice

One of the major problems in categorising a birth as low risk or normal is that the precise definition of normal is elusive. Although normality is highly valued by midwives, they find it difficult to define (and measure). Our attempts to elicit what the participants meant by the term frequently met with laughter or expressions like *'Oh no!', 'I don't know', 'How am I supposed to answer that?', 'That's a difficult one'*; or even on one occasion, *'You can't expect me to be able to tell you that!'* (Extracts from interviews with midwives).

This inability to define normality was also evident in our interviews with a representative from the Royal College of Midwives (RCM). While discussing the impact of the College's *'Campaign for Normal Birth'* (Day-Stirk 2005, RCM 2010), the representative told us that, in the UK, midwives are so desensitised by over-use of the term 'normal birth' that it has become devoid of real meaning:

> We have had the normal birth debate such a long time in the UK, and people are quite …
> We are slightly blasé about it, and people, they sort of … they have had enough. I mean if I
> talk to a UK midwife about normal birth, they say, 'Well what's that? What's normal to
> you was not normal to us and does it mean anything at all anymore in the context of
> modern obstetrics?' It is almost as if it is, I don't know, kind of a nothing, if you like.
> (Extract from interview with representative)

At the same time as viewing normal birth as desirable, the midwives who participated in this study struggled to conceptualise it as a concrete concept. Rather, it was frequently described as something that could only be defined in terms of the absence of other more tangible attributes. More specifically, normality was something that revealed itself through the absence of risk indicators or specific risk management measures.

This definition by absence underpins the national 'Normal Birth Consensus Statement' in which normal birth is defined via a series of negatives as:

> Without induction, without use of instruments, not caesarean section and without general,
> spinal or epidural anaesthesia before or during delivery. (Maternity Care Working Party
> 2007)

This statement was developed, ironically, *'to encourage a positive focus on normal birth'* (Maternity Care Working Party 2007, p. 2). However, the choice of wording in this statement renders normal birth without substance. Instead, it is only present as a linguistic absence.

Given this wider context, it is not surprising that the majority of midwives who participated in this study saw normal birth in terms of what it was not, as an absence rather than a presence. For example, one midwife defined normal birth in the following way:

> Yes, I mean normal birth is a labour that has had minimal intervention, I mean medical
> intervention, no medical intervention, yer no medical intervention. That includes epidural.
> (Extract from interview with Rachael, midwife)

Another midwife described normality in terms of a negative tick list, the absence of a series of complications:

Well even now, I still do it. I, I go through it and, you know, the woman's pushing, and I'm like, 'Okay, is this all normal?' 'Yep we've got not foetal distress; we've got no problem with the woman's observations; erm' she has got this far and there is nothing'. It is almost like a tick-list in my mind ticking-off ... There is nothing [abnormal], *so it must be normal.* (Extract from interview with Hannah, an independent midwife)

In these discussions, normal birth was *'the subject that is not one'* (Butler 1999, p. 2). In midwifery conversation, normality has no language of its own. It has to be defined against the dominant discourse of high risk (Kress 1989) which invokes the language of pathology and medical intervention. There were no words with which to police the boundaries of normality, no linguistic tools to protect its integrity. Normality could only be signified through absence within the privileged discourse of risk.

The absence of normality not only was evident in midwives' talk, but could also be detected in the official texts designed to structure their practice, and in practice itself. For example, the Midwives Rules and Standards (Nursing and Midwifery Council 2004) define the legal framework for midwifery practice. These rules and standards delineate the midwifery 'care' **without any explicit reference to normality**, defining midwife care as:

preventative measures, the detection of abnormal conditions in mother and child, the procurement of medical assistance and the execution of emergency measures in the absence of medical help. (Nursing and Midwifery Council 2004, p. 36)

All four of the midwifery activities listed by the Council coalesce around the language of risk. According to the statutory regulative body, midwifery activity has nothing to do with normality. Rather, it is about detection and prevention of risk: being alert to the possibility of problems; accessing medical support in order to manage risk; and being capable of managing unexpected crises while medical assistance is sought.

It is therefore hardly surprising that our observations of midwifery practice showed that midwives were on the constant look-out for abnormality and risk. Midwives routinely 'manage' the birthing process by measuring vital signs of both the mother and baby, and monitoring 'progress' in labour – assessing uterine contraction and cervical dilatation. At the point when labour was identified, midwives initiated detailed surveillance and record keeping. Such intensive monitoring was applied to both normal/low risk and abnormal/high risk births, bringing all labouring women into visibility. The midwives involved in this study introduced this surveillance in a taken-for-granted manner. Its precise purpose was rarely made explicit to the birthing mother. Rather, each intervention was introduced as part of the customary care plan, the purpose of which was treated as self-evident. Midwives commonly introduced monitoring activities with comments like:

*'I'm **just** going to have a listen in again now, **just** to make sure the baby is okay'. This* preceded exposing the woman's abdomen to auscultate the foetal heart (Extract from field notes GT 20, author's emphasis) or *'Can I have your arm a minute. I need to check your blood pressure'.* (Extract from field notes RS1, authors' emphasis)

Underpinning these mother–midwife interactions was the implicit assumption that repeated checking, rechecking and recording of parameters such as fetal heart and maternal blood pressure were beneficial in terms of risk management. Once the measurements were taken, they were plotted in the partogram,[6] and/or written into the labour care section of the maternal notes. These measurements become central to the categorisation of risk, with normality indicated by the absence of signs of abnormality:

> *I suppose* [normality is] *no intervention. Just letting the woman listen to her body and do it herself, yer ... And well, you know, when everything is in the normal parameters; making sure, erm, like keep the woman and baby safe by making sure, you know, you are listening in every 15 minutes and that they don't come out the brackets thing, the chart thing ... partogram.* (Extract from interview with Harriet, a student midwife).

The midwives' talk to pregnant women following these measurements was generally quite cheerful. However, this approach did not always allay the fears that surveillance seemed to introduce, as the following extract from the field notes suggests. Sarah, a first time mother, was undergoing a routine vaginal examination to measure the dilatation of the cervix and descent of the baby's head.

> During the examination the room went very quiet. Sarah is lying flat on the bed as instructed by the midwife. No explanation is given to explain why this is necessary and no attempt is made to perform the examination in a position that might be comfortable for Sarah. It is as if any concerns for Sarah's physical or emotional comfort seem to be temporarily suspended given the seriousness of the task of finding out what is going on. The findings of the exam are not mentioned during the procedure, Sarah and her partner are left wondering and waiting, there is a palpable sense of tension. Afterwards Pauline [the midwife] explains what she found. Both parents look anxious and although the VE[7] shows progress of the labour was normal, both Sarah and her partner needed to repeatedly have this confirmed. Pauline did not seem surprised by this reaction, she smiled and reiterated that everything was fine at least three times. She then left the room to record her finding in the notes and on the board. (Extract from field notes PS 14)

In this case, Sarah's labour was following the desired partogram trajectory – she had progressed according to the parameters set by the chart. Although normality was confirmed, the process introduced a sense of uncertainty. Before the examination, both Sarah and her partner had been managing the labour process effectively and pretty much independently. But when the time came to monitor the progress, to check for normality or more precisely to hunt for abnormality, their confidence in the process and their understanding of the active role they could play in that process seemed to dissipate. Indeed, although Pauline, the midwife, stressed that progress was good, Sarah responded by asking '*Is there anything else I should be doing. Am I doing it right?*' (Extract from field notes PS14). Even when a woman's labour fits within the partogram trajectory, the very process of monitoring progress simultaneously confirmed and disturbed normality.

Through the action of routine surveillance, midwifery activity was oriented not to confirming normality, but to searching for the absence of abnormality. This was a subtle but significantly different task which tended to privilege imagined possibilities of 'what if things go wrong', and thereby operated to unsettle a woman's confidence in her body's ability to birth her baby successfully. Although midwives wanted to reassure mothers, their actions tend to expose the unstable base on which understandings of normality rest, as well as the unarticulated issue of accountability if anything went wrong. The labouring woman and her birthing partner were far from oblivious to this instability. As the above quotation illustrating Sarah's need for professional reassurance suggests, parents could and did easily recognise the midwife's concern with the ever-present 'virtual risk object' (Van Loon 2002, Heyman *et al.* 2010).

Discussion

The categorisation of a birth as low or high risk had important consequences for the ways in which it was managed. Categorisation as low risk enabled a normal midwife-supervised birth to be initiated, whereas placing a birth in the high risk category triggered increased surveillance and medical intervention. Midwives treated 'normal' birth as a self-evident good. But, because they were unable to define and measure normality, this categorisation was always tentative, and based on a provisional absence of risk indicators. Because the midwives who participated in our study found it hard to describe, talk about and measure normality and low risk, they effectively created an imagined future colonised by potential high risk that could at any moment be made visible through their continual surveillance.

Normality was absent from both official prescriptions about midwifery practice and midwives' talk. This absence is not just semantic, which would be disturbing enough given the moral loading of the term in midwifery talk. It is absolute.[8] As we noted, the Nursing and Midwifery Council's Midwives Rules and Standards require midwifery activity to focus on imagined futures where the possibility of pathology is ever-present, at the expense of the mostly much more probable alternative future inhabited by normality. This precautionary approach to risk management disregards the probabilities of events and '*casts the future principally in negative, potentially catastrophic terms*' (Alaszewski and Burgess 2007, p. 349). As Heyman *et al.* (2010, pp. 22–24) have argued the answer to the question of contingency, i.e. 'What might happen' is 'Absolutely anything!'. The data presented in the present paper show how midwives selectively populate the infinity of possibility with what might go wrong. This interpretive lens is shaped by the organisational and wider culture in which they operate and discounts the small magnitude of most of the relevant probabilities.

Furthermore, the inability to articulate and defend normal or natural birth provides the basis of the blame culture within midwifery. As Douglas and Wildavsky (1982, p. 35) have argued:

> *Blameworthiness takes over at the point where the line of normality is drawn. Each culture rests upon its own ideas of what ought to be normal or natural. If a death is held to be normal, no-one is blamed.*

The challenge for midwives is that, despite their efforts and commitment, 'blame-free' birth does not exist. All births are supervised by experts, and when something goes wrong, a search and inquiry starts to identify who and what is to blame. This organisational context provides the context for midwife talk and practice.

Midwives working in the birthing environment contemplate two possible imagined futures. In one, the baby is born through the natural process of spontaneous delivery and unnecessary medical interventions pose an unacceptable risk of iatrogenic harm. In the other, nature fails, threatening the health of mother and/or baby, and serious harm might occur without timely intervention involving technological procedures. Importantly, both of these imagined futures are value-laden, with the former considered by midwives as the most desirable to both mother and midwife (Newburn 2006). As the evidence presented suggests, the latter, although less desirable, represents the more persuasive of the two imagined futures within the current birthing climate. In this climate, caesarean section rates have risen sharply, both nationally (Mander 2008, NHS Information Centre 2009) and globally (World Health Organization 2009); and 97% of women end up giving birth within a hospital environment 'just in case' (Devries *et al.* 2001, NHS Information Centre 2011b). As Murphy-Lawless (1998, p. 21) has pointed out, this anxiety about risk not only disempowers both midwives and birthing mothers:

> The tendency has ... increasingly been to define every aspect of pregnancy and birth in terms of risk in a mistaken attempt to cover all possible eventualities. In this sense, the entire female body has become risk-laden.

Conclusion

In this article we have shown how the categorisation of risk shapes, and is shaped, by the social context for decision-making. As normality lacks any language of its own through with which midwives can defend its boundaries, it is easily subsumed by the linguistically and culturally more secure notion of risk. Through the analysis of published texts and midwifery activity, we have shown how midwives create an **ever closing window of normality** in which all births are categorised as risky. Within a linguistic context where normality and unassisted safety could only be envisaged as the non-occurrence of unwanted futures, imagined futures where things go wrong took on a very real existence in the present, thereby impacting upon how birth could be conceptualised and managed. As such, midwifery activity functions not to preserve normality, but to introduce a pathologisation process where birth can never be imagined to be normal until it is over.

Notes

1. This section provides only a brief descriptive account of methods. Detailed discussion of the methodological implications of the research design, in terms of author impact and construction of identity, translation of culture, sequential consent, etc., has been presented elsewhere and is beyond the remit of this paper.
2. Ten midwifery managers, 10 midwives, two student midwives, two independent midwives and three pressure group representatives.
3. The first author is a registered midwife, but for the purposes of the study is licensed to practice as a maternity care assistant.
4. Stretch and sweep is a procedure where a midwife or doctor will 'sweep' a finger around the cervix during an internal examination. The aim is to separate the fetal membranes from the cervix, leading to a release of prostaglandins and subsequent onset of labour (National Institute for Health and Clinical Excellence 2008, p. xii).
5. Both interventions into the birth process are done by midwives without any recourse to the multidisciplinary team. These are what might be called midwifery interventions and, as such, are seen not as interventions at all, but as part of a process for facilitating normal birth (Annandale 1988).
6. The partogram, or picture of labour, is a universal chart designed in the 1970s for recording observations of mother and baby, including contraction pattern rate and strength, cervical dilatation, etc.
7. Vaginal examination.
8. The text being analysed here is the printed 2004 version. It should be noted that the online version has an update to include a more up-to-date International Confederation of

Midwives definition which does include reference to normality. The modality of this reference, however, is significantly reduced as the word is sandwiched between other risk-orientated concerns and appears in a list of five activities, four of which coalesces around risk and abnormality.

References

Alaszewski, A. and Burgess, A., 2007. Risk, time and reason. *Health, Risk & Society*, 9 (4), 349–358.

Annandale, E., 1988. How midwives accomplish natural birth: Managing risk and balancing expectation. *Social Problems*, 35 (2), 95–110.

Bryman, A., 2004. *Social research methods*. 2nd ed. Oxford: Oxford University Press.

Butler, J., 1999. *Gender trouble: Feminism and the subversion of identity*. London: Routledge.

Centre for Maternal and Child Enquiries, 2011. Saving mothers' lives: Reviewing maternal deaths to make motherhood safer: 2006–08. The eighth report on confidential enquiries into maternal deaths in the United Kingdom. *BJOG*, 118 (Suppl. 1), 1–203.

Clifford, J. and Marcus, G.E., eds., 1986. *Writing culture: The poetics and politics of ethnography*. Berkeley: University of California Press.

Confidential Enquiry into Maternal and Child Health, 2009. *Perinatal mortality 2007: United Kingdom*. London: CEMACH.

Davenport, R., n.d. *The relationship between stillbirth and early neonatal mortality: Evidence from eighteenth century*. London: Cambridge Group for the History of Population and Social Structure. http://www.geog.cam.ac.uk/people/davenport/davenport9.pdf.

Davis-Floyd, R., *et al.*, eds., 2009. *Birth models that work*. Berkeley: University of California Press.

Day-Stirk, F. 2005. The big push for normal birth. *RCM Midwives*, 8 (1), 18–20.

Denzin, N.K., 1998. The new ethnography. *Journal of Contemporary Ethnography*, 27 (3), 405–415.

Denzin, N.K., 2002. Confronting ethnography's crisis of representation. *Journal of Contemporary Ethnography*, 31 (4), 482–490.

Devries, R., *et al.*, 2001. What (and why) do women want? The desires of women and the design of maternity care. *In*: R. Devries, *et al.*, eds. *Birth by design. Pregnancy, maternity care and midwifery in North America and Europe*. New York: Routledge, 243–266.

Douglas, M., 1990. Risk as a forensic resource. *Dædalus. Journal of the American Academy of Arts and Sciences*, 119 (4), 1–16.

Douglas, M., 1992. *Risk and blame: Essays in cultural theory*. London: Routledge.

Douglas, M. and Wildavsky, A., 1982. *Risk and culture: An essay on the selection of technological and environmental dangers*. Berkeley: University of California Press.

Fairclough, N. and Wodak, R. 1997. Critical discourse analysis'. *In*: T. van Dijk, ed. *Introduction to Discourse Analysis*. London: Sage, 258–284.

Fairclough, N., 2001. *Language and power*. Harlow: Pearson Education Press.

Fairclough, N., 2003. *Analysing discourse: Textual analysis for social research*. London: Routledge.

Giddens, A., 1991. *Modernity and self-identity. Self and society in the late modern age*. Cambridge: Polity Press.

Gould, D., 2000. Normal labour: A concept analysis. *Journal of Advanced nursing*, 31 (2), 418–427.

Graneheim, U. and Lundman, B., 2004. Qualitative content analysis in nursing research: Concepts, procedures and measures to achieve trustworthiness. *Nurse Education Today*, 24 (2), 105–112.

Green, J., 1999. From accidents to risk: Public health and preventable injury. *Health, Risk & Society*, 1 (1), 25–39.

Gwyn, R., 2002. *Communicating Health and Illness*. London: Sage.

Heyman, B., *et al.*, 2010. *Risk, safety, and clinical practice health care through the lens of risk*. Oxford: Oxford University Press.

Kress, G., 1989. *Linguistic processes in sociocultural practice*. Oxford: Oxford University Press.

Leap, N., 2000. The less we do, the more we give. *In*: M. Kirkham, ed. *The midwife/mother relationship*. London: Macmillan.

Loudon, I., 1993. *Death in childbirth: An international study of maternal care and maternal mortality 1800–1950*. Oxford: Oxford University Press.

Malinowski, B., 1932. *Argonauts of the Western Pacific*. 2nd ed. London: George Routledge.

Mander, R., 2008. *Caesarean: Just another way of birth?* London: Blackwell Synergy.

Maternity Care Working Party, 2007. *Making normal birth a reality. Consensus statement from the maternity care working party our shared views about the need to recognise, facilitate and audit normal birth*. London: NCT, RCM and RCOG.

Menzies, I., 1960. Social systems as defense against anxiety: An empirical study of a nursing service of a general hospital. *Human Relations*, 13, 95–131.

Midwifery 2020 Team. 2010. *Midwifery 2020. Delivering expectations*. Cambridge: Midwifery 2020 Programme.

Murphy-Lawless, J., 1998. *Reading Birth and Death: A History of Obstetric Thinking*. Cork: Cork University Press.

National Institute for Health and Clinical Excellence, 2008–last update. *Induction of labour*. [homepage of RCOG, online]. Available from: http://www.nice.org.uk/nicemedia/pdf/ CG070FullGuideline.pdf [Accessed 2010].

Newburn, M., 2006. What women want from care around the time of birth. *In*: L. Page and R. McCandlish, eds. *The new midwifery. Science and sensitivity in practice*. 2nd ed. Philadelphia: Churchill Livingstone, 3–20.

NHS Health and Social Care Information Centre, 2011a. Place of delivery. Available at http:// www.hesonline.nhs.uk/Ease/servlet/ContentServersiteID=1937&categoryID=1815 [Accessed February 2012].

NHS Information Centre, 2011b. Maternity Data 2010 – 2011 Available at http://www. hesonline.nhs.uk/Ease/servlet/ContentServersiteID=1937&categoryID=1815 [Accessed February 2012].

Nursing and Midwifery Council, 2004. *Midwives rules and standards*. Professional rules and standards ed. London: Nursing and Midwifery Council.

Reissman, C., 1993. *Narrative analysis. Qualitative research methods series 30*. London: Sage.

Rosser, J., 1998. Fools rush in … how little we know about normal birth. *The Practising Midwife*, 1 (9), 4–5.

Royal College of Midwives, 2010. *Campaign for normal birth* [homepage of Royal College of Midwives, online]. Available from: http://www.rcmnormalbirth.net/ [Accessed January 2010].

Sandall, J., *et al*., 2009. Discussions of findings from a Cochrane review of Midwife-led versus other models of care for childbearing women: Continuity, normality and safety. *Midwifery*, 25, 8–13.

Silverman, D., 1988. *Communication and medical practice: Social relations in the clinic*. London: Sage.

Silverman, D., 2004. *Qualitative research: Theory, method and practice*. London: Sage.

Spradley, J., 1979. *The ethnographic interview*. New York: Holt, Rinehart and Winston.

Spradley, J., 1980. *Participant observation*. New York: Holt, Rinehart and Winston.

The Health and Social Care Information Centre, 2009. *Maternity: Key facts, 2008–09*. London: The Health and Social Care Information Centre.

Van Dijk, T., 1993. Principles of critical discourse analysis. *Discourse & Society*, 4 (2), 249–283.

Van Dijk, T., ed., 1997. *Discourse as structure and process*. London: Sage.

Van Loon, J., 2002. *Risk and technological culture: Towards a sociology of virulence*. London: Routledge.

Wagner, M., 1994. *Pursuing the birth machine*. Camperdown: Ace Graphics.

Wodak, R., 1999. Introduction: Organizational discourse and practices. *Discourse and Society*, 10 (5), 5–18.

World Health Organization, 2009. *Monitoring emergency obstetric care*. France: WHO Library Cataloguing-in-Publication Data.

Index

Milton Keynes UK
Ingram Content Group UK Ltd.
UKHW051854071024
449327UK00025B/1953